MY PINK CHOICE

CAROL KILPATRICK

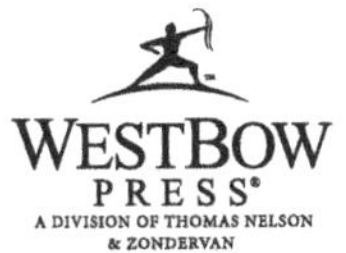

WestBow Press books may be ordered through booksellers or by contacting:

WestBow Press
A Division of Thomas Nelson & Zondervan
1663 Liberty Drive
Bloomington, IN 47403
www.westbowpress.com
844-714-3454

ISBN: 979-8-3850-3529-8 (sc)
ISBN: 979-8-3850-3530-4 (hc)
ISBN: 979-8-3850-3531-1 (e)

Library of Congress Control Number: 2024920955

Print information available on the last page.

WestBow Press rev. date: 12/05/2024

For John, Andrew, Kristen, MacKayla,
Cara, and Lily, my village

Contents

Prologue

I lost my identity when I faced the difficulty of navigating breast cancer. Any space to be genuine was choked out by the demands of the disease, the urgency of care, and the sudden looming fear over my life. I was forced to surrender my personality, my interests, my freedom, and many choices. The disease demanded my entire focus, attention, and energy as my individuality shifted solely to someone I no longer recognized. I was powerless, unprepared, and removed as I felt helpless to do anything but watch it happen. As I lost control, I wondered if my true self would ever reappear.

When this journey started, I knew nobody with cancer and had no experience, no heads-up, and no warning. I searched for resources and was desperate not to feel alone. I longed for connection, for understanding, and for warning about everything that would be interrupted in my life. While searching for help, navigating, and processing emotions, I realized a void in support and resources. I became inspired to use my story to help others attempting to leap over the same daunting familiar hurdles.

Learning you have cancer causes shock, dismay, and betrayal that you feel in your own body when you are faced with the surprising news of such a diagnosis. I desire to connect with, encourage, inspire, and be a friend to those who find themselves somewhere along this journey. Cancer affects many people, and if it is not you, it will likely be someone you know in your lifetime. Assuredly, I am not the only one ever to have lost heart and wondered how such a journey would end. I hope you find a place to connect and feel partnered with, understood and validated on your journey.

Equally, I hope the people around you understand your needs, support how you feel, and contribute to your overall health and well-being. Overcoming challenges and thriving through challenging times requires love and support. I realize that dealing with cancer is already overwhelming, and taking on the responsibility of communicating a patient's needs to a caregiver adds another significant challenge. I hope this information is insightful, especially for those learning to fulfill the role of a caregiver and play a crucial part in a cancer patient's support system as an essential part of their "village."

I have never been much for journaling, but when I was submerged in this overwhelming season, I began to write down what happened, how it felt, and how it affected my life. It has taken me ten years to compile my writings and unpack the profound ripple cancer caused across my life. This story was written to help anyone who has been affected by cancer understand what it feels like for those it touches. As I recount the details, I invite you to join me in experiencing my journey firsthand and gain insight into the messy, unpredictable devastation that cancer produces.

I choose to pour out with simplicity an honest account of all this disease has cost me, with the belief that what I share can bring understanding, healing, and hope to someone else. My desire to openly funnel my personal story is a result of my collected losses. I am choosing to share and offer insight specifically into the emotions involved, because the space to understand and work through these emotions may be limited or nonexistent. Emotions, the ones we tend to stuff or think we can skip, must be confronted honestly. It is still a challenge for me to find words that hold enough meaning to relay the impact of this season. I continue because I do not want to selfishly hold onto any part of this experience that could provide the necessary insight and support that someone facing cancer longs for.

Throughout these pages, I have chosen to omit the long medical terms, my own specifics, and the names of the many medicines used to treat cancer. *My Pink Choice* is not about the technicalities of the disease or its treatments. It is about the personal journey, the emotional roller coaster, and the heart issues that come along with receiving a cancer diagnosis and the associated treatments for the diseases. It is about our shared experiences and the understanding that comes from walking this unknown path.

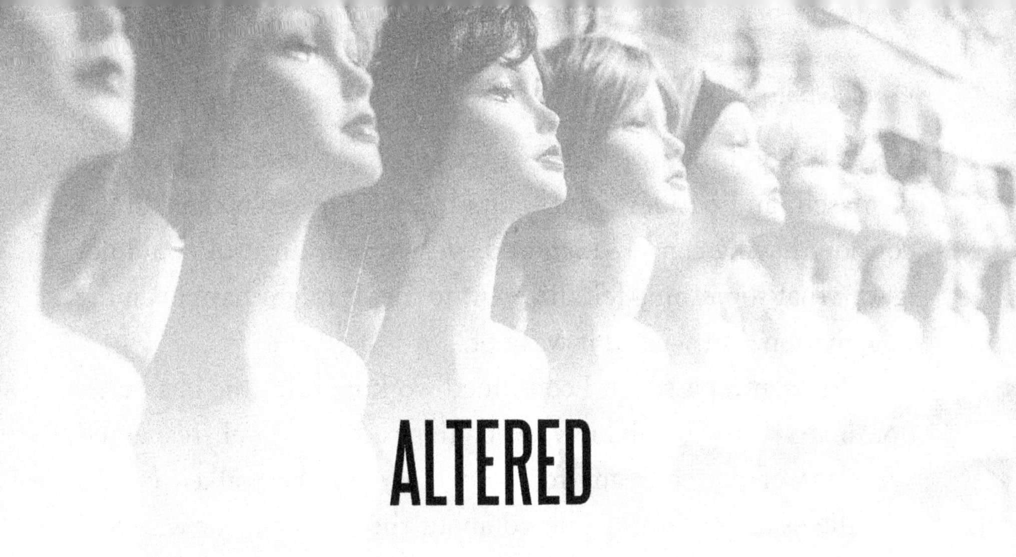

ALTERED

As I begin writing this story, my hair, the most obvious sign to me of time passing, is down to the middle of my back. A lot has happened, and a lot has changed. I have navigated the disruption to my life caused by a breast cancer diagnosis. It has been two long and challenging years since I put aggressive treatments behind me. I began to look through my journal. I am on the other side, and I realize I am no longer the same as I was when all this started.

I had one other mammogram in my life a few years before the cancer diagnosis. I was following the recommended schedule for getting checked now that I had reached my midforties. The mammogram was routine and uncomfortable but uneventful. Afterward, I quickly dismissed the appointment. Not knowing what to expect, I expected nothing. I mentally checked the box and was proud of myself for completing the test, but I never gave it another thought.

Four years later, it was October, Breast Cancer Awareness Month. Everywhere I looked I saw advertising reminders to get checked, and I worked to ignore all of them. I had been sensing this urge to get my second mammogram, but with every thought that arose, I matched it with an excuse. Time, cost, hassle, inconvenience, unnecessary worry, embarrassment, pain. As a busy wife and mom, I had an excuse for not taking better care of myself, and besides, who wants to make space in their life to consider having cancer? I ignored every prompting but could not ignore that something felt different to me. It might have been my imagination, but what if it was not?

The month passed as I continued working full time in a male-dominated office. I had worked alongside the well-respected president of the company for years. One day he walked in and casually asked me if I had heard about the news anchor who had been given the assignment to do a story on mammograms. "She was hesitant," he said. "She had never had one before." He went on to finish. "She reluctantly agreed to participate in her own first screening, and with the cameras rolling, they found advanced-stage breast cancer."

I had been unusually distracted by the topic as I had been noticing advertisements for breast cancer for the past month. This became the last obvious hint that I could not ignore. "OK, I get it," I quietly said to myself, "I'll finally make an appointment." And I did.

I was in between doctors then, so I contacted a new gynecologist's office and made the appointment. "Do you feel a lump?"

"No," I answered casually. "No rush for an appointment. I can wait until you can fit me in." I got off the phone with more concern than I wanted to confront and privately wondered where this was going.

Something did not feel right to me. I felt unusually patient and apprehensive at the same time. Nevertheless, I was willing to wait in line for my turn to be seen. I focused on the fact that I had now taken the necessary steps toward the screening and pushed every related thought out of my mind.

Two weeks had passed, and here I was at what became the beginning of this medical journey. Since I was a new patient, I was unfamiliar with how their office and testing procedure worked and did not know what to expect. I received a routine exam, and everything seemed to be status quo. "We call a certain percentage of people back. Do not be alarmed if we call you. We may just want another look," I was told as I put my clothes back on. I left hoping I would never see or hear from them again, unsure if this was even a doctor I would want to keep.

A few days later, on a Friday afternoon, I received a call-back message. The doctor's office and I played phone tag until the end of business the following Monday. I learned that another look would be necessary in my case. They quickly fit me into their schedule a few days later. And I continued to keep this mysterious appointment to myself. I decided there was no real reason to share that I had been called back. This was only a protocol path, and it may or may not have meant anything.

As I sat pondering where I was and casually reading through health magazines in the waiting room, I wondered if there were any pieces I could put together yet.

Back again. Twice in less than a week. *Let us please get this second look over quickly*. It was apparent to me, in hindsight, that the nurse at that second appointment had known the diagnosis long before I saw it coming. She was oddly awkward as she led me around the maze of chairs, past the strong smell of burnt coffee, and through the doors, laughing a little too nervously.

I was in a patient gown and already feeling more vulnerable than relaxed. Her mannerisms were quirky, and I thought it odd that she would not look me in the eye. Same routine, different day, and not much of an explanation. "We really cannot say."

"We really are not sure."

"There is nothing we can tell you."

"The radiologist will have to call you." This was the first mention of a radiologist being officially looped into my care. I was slightly curious and surprised at the casual leap that had just happened with that statement.

The radiologist called, and I was immediately referred to the next stage for a biopsy of what they saw. The brief conversation, which clearly had been rehearsed, was limited and direct. There was no room to ask questions that were not already being answered from a basic script.

"We also want you to meet with a surgeon soon, just in case."

That seems unnecessary, I thought. Again, another giant leap in this situation happened right before me.

"We want you to have a surgeon in place in case you need one."

What? Why? Really? I thought. I had more questions than anyone wanted to answer honestly at that stage. No more details were given, but it was said to me, "We are being cautious." It was Friday afternoon again, and the upcoming weekend already felt overwhelmingly long to face considering this unexpected heavy exchange.

I am now backed into a corner. It is the first time I must share this important thing that is happening to me. I am not prepared, and I am still trying to unpack the past few days. I have no idea how you need to hear it, how I need to say it, or how my telling you a certain way could help either of us. I pick you up from work, and after a short greeting, I begin the familiar drive home. After driving a short distance, I blurt out that I had a bad mammogram. I do not have many answers, and your list of questions is longer than my short interaction with the radiologist on the phone.

You ask me repeatedly if I am kidding. I understand; this is unfair and sounds wild enough to be made up, but I would never kid around about something like this. I am sorry and wish I could undo telling you, because you are visibly distraught by my news. I cannot promise you what I do not know myself, and trying to promise anything seems fruitless.

We drive home the rest of the way mostly in silence. There is nothing else to say and nothing else worth talking about. There are no words. I feel sure that my news just drastically changed our lives.

And that was how I told my husband that the doctors suspected I had breast cancer.

Separately, he and I become focused researchers and students of cancer, learning about the many types, stages, symptoms, treatments, prognoses, and remedies—anything to help us get a handle on this current situation. We waited and we walked, and when we felt strong enough, we did our best to push away the subject and all our concerns. We often lied to ourselves about our feelings and how this was affecting us. It was not easy. There was no part of our lives that the idea of cancer did not begin to overshadow. We were of little help to each other, a situation that went on for weeks while we waited for more answers and for the next appointment to arrive.

I met with the surgeon—a nice guy—but it was not much of an appointment. The nurse asked me to dress in a paper gown, and I secretly hoped he would come in and do a quick exam and clear up what may have been a misunderstanding. We met, but neither of us had any solid information. He was older and easy to relate to. I pictured him as a grandpa and a family man.

What was potentially happening was buried deep in my cells. And there were no visible signs to check for. I sat there, and it seemed unreasonable that I was dressed in this gown because there was no physical exam.

"We'll see what the results are from the biopsy," the surgeon said. This was clearly intended as a meet and greet disguised as an essential exam. We had now met, so that requirement was done.

Optimistically, I hoped there would be no second appointment. I mentally checked that box and kept moving.

Two more weeks passed, and we were now in another new office, waiting on a different doctor to do the biopsy. I liked her—I liked the nurse. They made the start of this serious appointment casual, simplistic, and unattached to any prognosis that was not positive. The lights were dimmed, and the small room was tranquil. The only sound was instruments being unwrapped and metal trays rolling across the floor.

I lay down on the sterile bed and settled in. A glaring domed light was adjusted and fixed above my head. An ultrasound was softly beeping on the monitor. I was injected in the breast multiple times with a long needle filled with numbing medicine. There was no room for conversation other than "Yes, I am fine," and "No, it doesn't hurt." Of course it hurt—it was a needle in my breast. But just in case this was not all I would have to endure, I chose to say bravely, "I am fine."

As I watched, another thick, hollow needle was injected repeatedly into what I would later learn was a tumor against my chest wall. I was doing my best to be patient, but I was a few additional restless weeks into this process, and I still knew nothing about what was happening in my body. I had no concrete information, and the questions and uncertainty in my mind had been mounding for too long.

Both women were serious, extremely focused, and working harmoniously. I was incredibly grateful at this moment that they were women. I imagined they must have been sensitive like me, and understanding, and must have known what being here and walking through this process felt like. So many injections with the needle. Nothing distracted me from watching them work and wondering what they were thinking. The room was too quiet. The only interruptions were them checking to see if I was doing OK and was comfortable.

My breast was fully numb. I felt no physical pain at this point, only mental anguish. Their voices and mannerisms were steady, professional, and extra kind. I could easily deduce in the time that went by and the intense tone of their work that what they were looking at was not good.

I was a moment away from knowing and honestly had no idea how I would react. *When I ask, and if they answer, there will be nowhere to escape.* I prepared myself and waited until I was ready to learn the truth. In a flash of courage, I broke the silence and strategically and carefully asked, "Is this something the surgeon will want to take out?"

There was a brief pause, and the doctor replied, "You seem like someone who wants the facts."

"Yes," I replied, thinking, *Yes, that is who I am.*

"Yes, he will," she said steadily and plainly, and it was over just like that. The moment before, I knew it was cancer, and the moment after, when life surrounding me was now altered. There was no disguising it or pretending they had not found what they had. It simply looked like it was cancer. It was time to adjust to this new reality that was about to stun my predictable life.

We went back to silence as the doctor and nurse continued with the biopsy. I noticed they did not exchange glances when I asked my question. I wondered, if they had, would they have found tears in each other's eyes? They were trained for this moment of diagnosis, but I wondered how it felt. Cancer, the thing they were skilled at spotting, was still not found in every case. When found, did it feel as tremendous to the one who must identify it as it did to the one who waited anxiously to hear?

I asked the doctor if she considered continuously passing the needle through the area until the mass was gone. She gave little attention to my words and continued the procedure. But I had been serious and thought my plan should be considered. Could it be taken out as simply as that? Once I realized there were cancer cells in my body, I did not want to leave them in there for another minute. I wanted a choice in this plan, wanted my plan to be listened to, and yes, wanted the doctor to explain to me if it was not a good one.

The doctor and nurse are wrapping up as I hear the doctor state, "I got everything I need for the lab." They break the tension once again with small talk.

Last, the doctor explains she will be inserting a small titanium marker in the shape of a swish into my breast, which I had no idea was even a thing. I was told it was happening as if it were routine. I had no other titanium pieces in my body. There was no routine here for me. The doctor explained that the marker would determine how the surgeon would find the lump. Who thought of this idea that seems so bizarre to me? If another company paid enough money, would the doctor have placed its logo inside me instead? I did not want to advertise this awful disease through any method, including the marker now inside me, however helpful it may have been to the process.

My husband sat unsuspecting in the waiting room, shoes off, magazine in hand, randomly reading whatever he could find. His female coworkers repeatedly reassured him that this appointment was nothing. "She got called back," he desperately confided.

"She'll be fine; this happens all the time," he had been carelessly told day after day. I did my best to continually remind him that things already were not fine. I had this feeling, and they did not know me. I asked him not to accept these comments as the conclusion and to please not carry such false hope coming from people I barely knew. The doctor retrieved my husband from the waiting area and brought him back to her office to deliver the news.

When it was over, I was taken to an oversized dressing room and helped into my clothes as my bra was packed with ice. The procedure nurse handed me aftercare instructions, reassured me, and sent me on my way. A little disoriented from all that had just happened, I found my way back to the waiting area and to my husband. I was unaware he had been told, and he was unaware I had found out. Neither of us had much to say as we watched each other looking for a sign. I noticed an underlying expression of deep sadness on his face. I knew he knew, but I was not sure how. He was wrecked, and this was the last place I wanted to be when it was time for us to unpack this thing that was now happening.

WHOLE

We tried to go back to our regular lives and waited three long days to get the results from the biopsy. I had been anxious all day at work, expecting a call from the same surgeon I was hoping never to encounter again. I received the long-awaited phone call in the afternoon. I stepped away from my desk and began to pace outside as we exchanged greetings.

"I am surprised, but it is cancer, and we need to take it out," he said in a direct and methodical way. The word *cancer* hit me hard as the official diagnosis sank in. At that point, I had already mentally prepared myself as best as I could for that particular outcome.

I was equipped with my answers just in case, but this was still surreal. I was running on autopilot. "It is small and caught early," the doctor said. "You probably won't even need chemotherapy, maybe just a little radiation."

A little radiation sounds harmless, I thought. I relayed that I wanted the cancer out as fast as possible and that I did not want to lose a breast. We had a short conversation about the facts and agreed that, in this case, it was appropriate to have only the lump removed. I was in a hurry to get the surgery done. I thought the faster we could get the mass out, the faster I would be cancer-free and put this all behind me. This part of the journey moved quickly, and I had determined to have it do just that. We set up another appointment and the surgery for the next open day on his calendar a few weeks later and a few days before Christmas.

After the next appointment, my husband and I would begin to tell the kids. We needed a plan. I needed a game face, but I did not have one. I was completely unprepared for all that I anticipated would be next, unable to imagine what to say, how to begin, or what to include. I could only go for a few seconds without showing the stress or uncertainty that this was causing. I used a blank stare a lot. I did not mean to, but I really did not have answers to anyone's questions—or mine. I was exhausted beyond what I had ever known and felt vacant and lost. How would I last through these conversations? How would I get the words out without my voice cracking? I had no assurance for anyone. I needed assurance myself.

I went back to the surgeon's office for the presurgery appointment. There was no mention of an exam this time. He was serious and a bit rushed, focusing on the instructions he had walked into the room to deliver. I was watching and listening to this happen as if my life had become a movie, wondering what was next, and I had no idea how it would end.

Look me in the eye. I don't just want to be your fifth appointment of the day or your eighth lumpectomy this month. Before you say anything else life-altering about me or my body, I want you to understand who I am, my whole story. Shouldn't you know some important things if you are about to take my life into your hands?

As a wife, mother, daughter, and sister, I am resourceful, creative, spontaneous, and instinctively entrepreneurial. I am also an overachiever and a perfectionist; I strive too hard not to miss anything; and I can be harder on myself than anyone else can.

I never saw this coming and cannot find the brakes to stop this whole situation—which makes me feel like I am no longer whole.

How does anyone handle this? I need to think. Cancer. Cancer! Cancer? I left the appointment with a six-page full biopsy report with details I did not understand. Could the labs have been wrong? Many people had signed off on these, and there were several numbers, terms, and measurements. There was a managing lab physician's name at the bottom. I had never met him. Was he sure? I wondered if he gave the results a second thought, wondered who I was, and considered how these results would change my life. Did he have a mother or an aunt with breast cancer? I had heard lab results could be wrong sometimes. Wrong labs probably did not look like this, did they? There were so many checks and balances on these pages. I was amazed at how many different terms and methods they used to describe this small (almost microscopic) cell group in my body. Why didn't I know it was there? There was no obvious sign. I could not feel it. I did not feel sick. I wondered how this happened, why, and what I had done wrong. I had so many questions at this point. I felt that I was out of options and was done trying to figure this out.

The oldest two kids were in college, finals were coming up, it was right before Christmas, and this was such an unfair time to drop such a distracting news bomb. I struggled with them one by one, sharing the news, answering their questions, and comforting their fears. I said the words alone repeatedly before trying to work my unsuspected update into a regular discussion with each of them.

I dodged the word *cancer* and instead described the treatment, cellular changes, and care plans. I talked my way around the hardest words for me to say and what I suspected would be the hardest for younger ears to hear. There was no upside at this point, but I did my best to put a positive spin on the information I shared. I had no idea if my optimistic method, words, or approach made any difference. All I could rely on was that God knew; He is the only one with any answers right now.

The other two kids went back and forth to their other parents' home. They were younger and walked away from their family support every time they left. Who would hug them and help them through this hurt? Who would care that they were concerned and sad? Who would answer their questions optimistically but honestly? How would they manage? This was too big for younger brains, and I hated that I was the source bringing it to them. There was no suitable time and no better way. I had to explain and reassure them in the same breath.

I processed so many feelings in the early days that my head felt that it was spinning with every piece of added information. I did not want to miss anything, so I tried my best to stay on top of the doctor's recommendations, my symptoms, side effects, and all the postrecovery information. It felt as if this new requirement had no end in sight and no satisfying result.

Nobody can think through that much that fast and for so long. I thought for hours until I was exhausted, and then hours again the next day. It was deep thinking combined with some intermittent crying and occasionally sobbing from a deep place of worry and anxiety over a wound I could not even feel or see. Nothing I thought through or figured out made it change or go away.

FAMILY

The big blue letters FAMILY hung above the entrance to our living room. Who could have thought that collecting this specific group of individuals with various needs balanced with talents would one day result in their complementing each other very well just like an orchestra perfectly combines instruments? Push, pull, give, take—life in unison with one another and all its many facets. God knew, and He had a plan that I did not see.

I have worked most of my professional career with young children. I am also focused on investing in my own children and believe children should be valued and raised respectfully with care and consideration. I am connected to my kids, both those in the house and those away at college, and these are genuine and good relationships.

Family is important to me. I have an empathetic heart for those who have not had the luxury of having sit-down family meals, gathering around a table, engaging in long talks, and sharing life with those with whom they share a name and a space. A sense of belonging is also important to me. Family should be the place you can always count on to fully experience that.

One afternoon, during Christmas break, my older kids watched a documentary about raccoons with me. They could have found something more interesting to do, but they did not. We sat there (me stretched out in discomfort after surgery) for an entire hour mindlessly watching animals play. We were all surprised by how entertaining it was, but more importantly, it was an hour I did not have to recover alone, an hour I got to forget why I was there. I was able to recoup some of the investment in these personal relationships that were so important and otherwise easily lost during that season. That increment of time was an hour closer to healing with a positive memory that overlapped the struggle.

It was time to tell the rest of our family. My sister taught mammography and had a great many questions, most of which I could only answer with, "I do not know." *I am in over my head,* I think, *and there is no way to catch up at this point.* At her request, I read her the report over the phone, including the descriptions and the numbers, and I listened intently to the tone of her replies. Nothing. She gave no sign, good or bad, of any of it. I had no idea what it was that I did not know or could learn.

I had other siblings and extended family. There were many people to include, and I had no choice but to keep moving forward. One by one, I did my best to inform each one and assigned some of them to tell others. I was moving through the steps with little ability to do anything but mentally check the boxes. I felt like a train crawling on the tracks, knowing that I could get derailed at any moment. All I was sure of was that this was such an unfamiliar territory, and I did not know where it was going.

When I called you to tell you I had cancer, I was already coping with it the best I could. I called you because I knew you loved me, and now we needed to add this to our relationship and begin to share this too. The timing, this being new and my not wanting to wait too long to tell you, made this conversation much harder. I was steady, and although you were ready to move our exchange to a different topic, I held on to the task at hand. "It probably is not cancer," you said to me.

I began to retell you all over again, helping you specifically hear what I had called you to say: "Yes, it is cancer."

Wow was the word you kept repeating. I realize now that your reaction was what it looks like when you are trying to cope. I had never seen you respond like this to anything with so few words. I had been digesting the news longer than you. You started telling me about treatments and cancer stories of other people you knew, doing your best to quote statistics from memory. When you kept summing it up for me, you meant no harm and were not disregarding me. You filled the conversation with your own various life updates and kept circling back to mine. You were trying to process and manage the news for yourself, and I needed to give you time to do so. By the time we passed along the typical sentiments and said our goodbyes, we were both drained.

"You are handling this so well"; "Your attitude is so good that I forgot you were sick"; "If I ever go through something like that, I hope I can handle it as well as you are." I collected these and similar comments in the back of my mind, never quite knowing how to give a response. How else could I have handled it? I did not remember the day when I was given a pass and told, "You do not have to participate." Also, I was not sick as I know sick to feel like. I think, *"Handling it very well." Is there another way? What does that mean, and what are the other options? This is my health and my body; I have only one, and it has already duped me once.*

I managed this moment by moment. I tried to think positively but lived with the looming idea that it could start all over again tomorrow. I internalized my thoughts and feelings and calculated when and where it was acceptable to let them out. Some days, I was not handling things well, but I showed an expressionless face and found that it was easier to keep my feelings on the inside rather than process honestly.

I wish you would ask me how I am really doing and refer to the cancer. I had spent a lot of time stuffing my thoughts and would appreciate an opportunity to unpack a few of them in a trusted place where I would not feel judged. My mind wandered a lot in directions you may not have suspected. I pondered what the lives of my children, husband, family, and friends would be without me, and I mentally processed my own early death. I considered the idea of not having the opportunity to turn old. I thought about if I would, or even could, do the treatments all over again. I wondered what a different choice would have brought. I speculated about the cancer coming back and told myself that if I let my guard down, it would come back.

I got distracted by pain, or by any twinge or swelling, and wondered if it could be a sign. I worried, but since I was trying not to, I hardly brought it up. I felt guilty when I talked about any of it. I was the one who added this pain to my family members' lives, and I really did not want to be the one to hurt any of them like that ever again.

I had surgery to remove the lump, along with seven lymph nodes from under my arm to check if the cancer had spread. Gratefully, it had not. The lab confirmed that it was an aggressive, fast-growing cancer that, thankfully, had been caught early. I went home to recover and do more lying around and healing during what should have been a busy holiday season, checking off lists, cooking, and planning.

A few days passed, and it was Christmas morning. Because I was getting dressed in my regular clothes for the first time since the surgery, I was beginning to assess the bandages and swelling and trying to find comfortable clothing to leave the house in. I had a small pillow I would need to keep tucked under my arm to compress the area where I had gotten stitches, which was tender and sore. There was no way to hide or not draw attention to the recent surgery site.

As I looked in the mirror for the first time, trying to figure it all out, I realized I now had two very noticeably different-sized breasts. The lumpectomy site had been described as small and I was not made aware that the result would be recognizable. Nobody thought to mention that this would be the outcome. Astonished, disappointed, and regretful, I realized I could do nothing about it now.

Our immediate family typically gathered for Christmas at our home on our acreage in Iowa with a big dinner, a tall tree, lots of homemade cookies, and made-up games. But this year was different. I could not make a meal or bake; there were none of our usual traditions or spontaneous fun; and I had no energy to help decorate the tree. I had to relinquish it all, knowing I could not manage the tiring cleaning and seasonal exhaustion that would follow every effort.

We were invited to my sister's house on Christmas, a day we would typically never leave our own house. She was considerate in trying to catch the pieces that would have been missing that year. We tried to push through the day and regain some normalcy, but nothing was normal. I was sore, tired, and sick from the aftereffects of the anesthesia. I spent the day uncomfortable, quietly trying to go unnoticed while making frequent trips to the restroom to be ill. What was missed that year was the peace, the family connections, the lighthearted silliness, and the details of our made-up traditions that always gave rise to the best memories.

I had two more weeks of healing and waiting until the next appointment, two more weeks of reassuring kids, sharing the scars, and taking medicine around-the-clock. Over the next few months, I walked through surgery to put the port in, chemotherapy, and surgery to take the port out, along with additional follow-up scans and appointments.

The port was an odd plastic protrusion from my chest near my heart, inserted just below my collarbone. The last thing I wanted was to have to explain this bandaged bulge, why it was there, or have anyone look at it instead of at me. The port was something I had never seen before or had any experience with. I was embarrassed by it and worked to find clothing to cover it. I could not manage unwelcome or hard-to-answer questions at this time, and I could not imagine a time when that would ever change.

Months after the surgery, I learned from my husband that when the surgeon removed the mass, he left staples inside me to forever mark the area where the tumor was. Staples? Really? Was there no better method than leaving common pieces of harsh metal behind? I swear, if I move wrong, I can feel them. Staples are not kind to skin; they are for paper. I added receiving staples to my mental list of choices lost and wondered if these things would always be part of my body.

Between the appointments and the recovery, we fit in other gatherings, family time, heart-to-heart talks, difficult phone calls, and many trips to the health food store searching for new supplements. I was tired, hurting, healing, and sometimes hopeless. I kept walking and trusted because it was all I could do. I had no experience, no point of reference, and no guidance from any other circumstance even close to this. I did not feel sick; I did not feel a lump; it did not add up; and I did not understand. Where had my former, predictable life gone?

I attended a graduation party with some family members and acquaintances I had not seen since this whole cancer journey had started. For me, there was no graduation from this situation. There was no comfortable way to navigate casual mingling or conversations. I stood there in my obvious wig that was dark and thick and that overpowered my face. I knew I did not look like me. I imagined my new look prompted an uncomfortableness that everyone was unprepared to navigate. Each time I hugged someone and their arm around me caught the back of my head, the wig shifted, and there was no discreet way to adjust it back. I felt embarrassed and internalized a situation I did not want or create.

Cancer is the first thing you asked me about now, and it was asked so casually and publicly without giving me the space to provide an honest answer. This was the new norm now. "How arrrrre youuuuu?" You stretched out the words, and it took me less than a minute to give an unreasonably brief update. I was living it out moment by moment, and it was taking too long. Several people later, I wondered if anyone had noticed I had switched my sincere answer to sarcasm.

When I explained some problematic parts of this process and you made it seem small, the reason I was telling you was that it felt big. Every appointment, every test, every day—the trivial things were now feeling Big. Only I reserved the right to blow them off, make them fit in a box, and treat them as minor. I was tired. I was aware that this was also affecting you, but please, listen more and give less advice. You were not there; even if you were, you are still not me.

Socializing or leaving the house for any extra purpose took a mental and physical strength I did not have. I did not want to be here or anywhere but the comfort of my home right now. I could not keep reassuring you through conversation; truthfully, I had no desire to find the energy to do so. Food smells bothered me, so I was uncomfortable going out somewhere when I did not know what to expect. Since the chemo treatment, I could no longer eat red meat because my stomach would ache for hours afterward. These experiences were new, uncomfortable, awkward, and unsuspectingly frustrating.

One of the many providers along the way mentioned I might have some aversion to foods after the chemo, but this was so much more and something for which I had not prepared. Chemotherapy kills every fast-growing cell in the body. Although you may be aware of common losses associated with it, there is more. You may not know that introducing certain foods again can also present a new challenge. Like a baby slowly learning to eat foods that are more difficult to digest, such as meat, I now was facing a new trial while also attempting to meet every vital nutritional goal.

I learned from my experience that in a case of cancer, most of the choices you may think you would have get taken away. Go here, pay for this, take that, schedule this, start that. Decisions begin to be made for you, not purposely to take your rights away, but because of past practice, proven history, best methods, statistics, and other pieces of the puzzle you know nothing about. You are unprepared for the most critical decisions in your life. They begin to be made for you, and you move through the maze of appointments, doctors, information, and schedules. Lost in the mix is what is important to you, your regular thoughts, and whatever your daily routine used to be. Forgotten is what you used to think were your biggest concerns, your usual focus, and your normal everyday family life.

CHEMO

Next, it was time to meet the oncologist. An appointment was made for me and I was sent to a new office in the same building, connected to the surgeon. The oncologist was armed with paperwork and explained she was new to the group and had just moved here from an oncology lab out of state. She was straightforward, blunt, and serious.

I had brought my husband and sister with me to catch some of the information I would inevitably miss. Medical terms, percentages of deaths and years of life, the drugs and their side effects, the procedures, and the risks—it was all part of this first appointment, and it was overwhelmingly long with too much content.

I wrote my signature on pages of forms giving my permission for the chemotherapy and acknowledging the risks and complications of the drugs. I signed every waiver, glancing through the fine print, but was far too overcome to consider trying to read or understand much of the technical jargon. I left with a stack of paperwork that I would never review again. This was the beginning of what became a thick cumulative medical file.

My husband and I went home, reeling from the details of the meeting. Functioning again on autopilot, we filled the seven prescriptions the doctor had written and began to take them according to schedule, while waiting to recover from the very recent lumpectomy surgery.

"Get your hair cut short." The oncologist's words hung in the air. "Cancer patients do not look good with hair missing in big clumps. In the second week after your chemo, it will begin to come out fast, and it will bother you more if it is longer." She continued, "You will find it on your pillow in the morning, and it will come out by the handful in the shower.

"Have a wig ready to go," she added. So direct, practical, and harsh all at the same time. I knew nothing about chemotherapy and had no idea its side effects were so precise and predictable. God was going to have to give me direction because I could not even think straight through all that was presented to me that day.

While I waited to start the chemo, I was feeling brave enough one day to try the recommended wig shop, conveniently located across the street from the cancer hospital. My husband and I walked in after a purposely planned lunch date in the same shopping center. I had never been a customer in a wig shop before and had no idea what to expect or the effect it was about to have on me. The long aisles were filled with hairpieces, hats, scarves, prosthetics, and medical gear displayed on row after row of expressionless mannequin heads. There were brands I was unfamiliar with, and hair replacement choices I had yet to learn would be a possibility. I did not last five minutes before I found my way quickly to the exit. "I am done," I told my husband in a panic, holding back tears I did not want to talk about. "I cannot do this." He somehow understood or felt the same way because we left without any further discussion about wigs that day.

A few weeks later, we took a second trip on a different day, walking in again and considering shopping for new hair. The salesperson, who had been there for twenty years, was across the street from the hospital and was used to a cancer story. She was kind, knowledgeable and compassionate, which made it easy for me to share my situation.

She assured me it usually took walking into this store a few times before feeling ready. She knew the inventory and the right questions to ask and was immediately aware of how to help, guiding me through the rows of white foam heads covered in every color and style imaginable.

As I began to learn about wigs, I discovered that they could be made of natural or synthetic materials and that the latter could melt in heat or get ruined in the rain. Real hair wigs must be shampooed and conditioned regularly and were expensive. Wigs for cancer patients, referred to as a "head prosthetic," could be obtained with a prescription from the doctor and were possibly covered by insurance. All wigs were at risk of slipping off suddenly and unexpectedly. The world of wigs was filled with lots to learn, and I had much to prepare and consider before I could make this new addition to my already changing daily routine.

I wanted a solution that would last with no possibility of "melting." I settled on a natural wig and was grateful that my insurance covered part of the cost. Natural wigs are made from hair typically grown and harvested in one part of the world, so they are available only in darker tones. That meant I could not find a wig that matched my natural color or texture, which had previously been straight, fine, and light to medium brown.

I chose a darker, full wig that was much coarser and thicker than I was used to. I put it on, and the stylist cut and shaped it like my former hairstyle. Despite my best selection and my being grateful to have natural hair, it was still not mine. When I wore it, I was self-conscious, and it always felt like I was wearing a costume.

The wig was hot and scratchy and often slipped around on my head, unbeknownst to me, yet obvious to others.

Nevertheless, the people who knew me never mentioned my updated hair, and those who did not know me had no idea that this was not my natural hair. Hiding that loss meant I could privatize how I felt about being bald, at least while I was in public.

At home, my family supported whatever I had on my head for the day. Everyone in my house saw my bald head sometimes, but since it was not very warm or comfortable, and because my hair had fallen out during the coldest months, it was common for me to keep my head covered with a soft hat. It was clear to me how I personally felt about being bald, but I had a plan and outwardly took it in stride.

My children took turns trying on my wig, and we laughed about how silly each of them looked. My husband surprised me by shaving his own head during this time. It was a nice gesture, and somewhere, we have a bald picture that we took together, but for me, it was no replacement for losing hair to cancer.

At my first appointment, this new oncologist entered the room with three cartoon-looking pages. On each page was a row of stick figures in dresses. It was unusually elementary considering the seriousness and what we were there to discuss. The first page, as she explained it to me, was representative of my life expectancy with only chemotherapy. I would gain the smallest number of years, depicted by the fewest stick figures in the row. The second page was representative of a lifespan with chemo plus radiation. The third page, with the most dressed stick figures, was representative of a lifespan with chemo, radiation, and ongoing medication.

In my case, I was told that a daily pill to block the hormones in my body, that had unknowingly fed the tumor, was the "highly recommended" course of treatment. There was no fourth page that diagrammed the probable loss of time for submitting my body to all those harsh chemicals, radiation, and medications. Nowhere represented in the picture or the conversation was the stress, sleeplessness, and emotional despair this was about to cause.

I sat there stuck, frozen, isolated, and quietly falling apart on the inside. I still remember the picture of a fairy-tale-like bridge that hung in the oncology office. I used to stare at the bridge and mentally check out while the doctor talked. I wished I could escape the medical terms she too casually used, run fast and far away from this place and this scenario I felt that I had been pushed into accepting.

Parts of the conversation that I wanted to have were being omitted. There was no discussion about my life and how it would be affected by the protocol she was discussing. I felt that I was in the dark and had lost any choice I thought I would have. This doctor knew nothing about me, my responsibilities, my values, or my concerns. Only God could help me manage the confusion and unease of the situation.

That daily recommended pill, which suppressed the ovaries, pushed the body into accelerated hormone changes, and altered physiology, was the only option explained to me. It affected my hormones responsible for mood, stress, weight, tiredness, sleeplessness, leg cramps, headaches, vision issues, etc.

In a different scenario, with a conversation where I was given an honest account of what taking that medicine would feel like, I could have been heard, valued, and still been made to feel like an individual. But no other choice was offered to me. The course was set, and I found myself automatically moving forward in a direction I was reluctant to follow.

In the beginning, I would rethink the idea of taking this medication versus not taking it daily. Bedtime: stand there with a glass of water in one hand and the pill in the other. It would have been much easier to drop the pill in the trash and run, forgetting everything. I secretly considered doing that many times.

Along with that one pill, I have learned to take various combinations of natural supplements to help curb some of the intrusive side effects—side effects that developed regularly and were seemingly without any foreseeable end. There was so much to process that I could have just sat down and fallen apart, but I could not afford to do only one thing.

Consequently, the medication had required too much troubleshooting over the years, and I did not find a combination that worked for more than just a brief period. I kept moving through the maze of appointments, doctors, recommendations, and expectations.

The most challenging hurdle for me was the effect the medication had on my sleep. I avoided bedtime because I found it difficult to stay asleep all night. I would wake up, and my mind would snap back to the reality of all that has happened and continued to unfold. Any feeling of restfulness quickly ended as the looming thoughts of cancer began all over again.

I do not know if I ever considered what chemotherapy was like before experiencing it myself. It was an unthinkable scenario filled with the darkest unknowns. I never had the opportunity to share much about the chemotherapy I went through. It was never part of the story anyone asked about, probably because it was unbelievable to imagine and unthinkable to ask a cancer patient to recollect.

For me, it was a collection of haunting moments and unforgettable observations that I am willing to share if they can give someone else firsthand insight.

My fragmented memories of chemotherapy are as follows:

I prepared to settle in for what I had been told would feel

like an eight-hour shift for the first dose of chemotherapy. I was anticipating what that day would bring but had no other similar experience or insight to prepare me.

Unexpectedly, I was led to a busy, overcrowded room filled with patients and IV poles. There were more patients than chairs. Bags of medicine were being hung and connected as I realized how many other people were also experiencing cancer.

Feeling suddenly overwhelmed and panicked by the entire situation, I asked for a quiet space, anywhere, to begin the treatments. The nurses honored my request, and my IV drip was started privately in a small exam room with just my husband.

Having the needle jabbed into the sensitive tissue around my very fresh and very sore port area for the first time and watching the medicine routed to my heart sickened me. Knowing some of what that medicine was about to cause sickened me and filled me with regret.

I was moved to the main room, my IV pole in tow, as the crowd thinned out and made space for the first-time or all-day-marathon patients. I was now fully aware that there was no turning back.

I was listening to the conversations of the other patients who had been going through this familiar treatment together for so much longer and wondered if their lighthearted comments reflected how they really felt and why this did not feel casual to me.

It was unsettling having the bags of medicine attached to the pole, one after the other, and understanding how lethal the drugs were that were streaming into my body. There was nothing else I could do but sit and wonder as the hours passed and I watched it happen.

Now that the port had been accessed, the nurse had to fish around in it with a needle under my skin, which both stung and was distressing to witness. I learned that the port was being used because the harsh medicines could otherwise destroy a vein in my arm.

Listening to the "frequent flyers" talk about medicine compounds, ordering lunch as if it were a matter of routine, and wearing attention-getting hats on bald heads. I could not imagine wearing a hat like that, viewing this experience as casual, or being a willing member of this club. I could not relate, which made me feel that I did not belong here.

There was no discrimination in this room. Cancer had seized the life of every person in there, those in wheelchairs, those in walkers, the young, and the old. I was somberly reminded that this rough season was also now a part of my story.

Sitting next to my husband, I began dozing off from the medicines while he held my hand and dozed off himself from pure exhaustion. I wondered what was going through his mind about being here in this place.

My sleep was disrupted by another medicine bag being changed, and I fully awoke to smiling nurses who had gathered to watch us from behind their desks. Hearing them mention they wished they had a camera made me realize plenty of patients were sitting all alone in there for their doses of chemotherapy.

I learned to read my husband's eyes and knew that sometimes when he walked out of the room with a legitimate excuse, he was really escaping so as not to lose his composure in front of me. Knowing my body, my health, and my diagnosis had caused him a great deal of fear, despair, and pain. I realized that nothing I could say would change that reality for him.

I walked out of chemotherapy with many serious discharge warnings but was unable to detect any physical changes it had presently caused in my body. The symptoms, laid out clearly, were serious and were oddly predicted to occur right on schedule.

I was at my lowest point sitting on the floor in our living room at home in front of a space heater hours after the chemo dose, trying to manage the bone pain in my legs and hips. Feeling dizzy, tired, sickened, bruised, unreasonably cold, and worn out, I wondered if this was the worst or if it would progress, and if so, how far it would go.

Hour by hour, I had pills to swallow on a strict schedule, keeping ahead of the pain, the nausea, the sleeplessness, and the anxiety. I realized there was no way I could do this without help, and I knew that some people had no alternative but to manage this alone.

I returned the following day to receive a painful shot to boost my immune system. It was intended to stimulate my body to regenerate the helpful red blood cells that had just been eliminated the day before. New intense side effects were again described and cautioned against.

In the aftermath, blisters and swelling rapidly reproduced in my mouth. There was concern about potential airway blockage with extra appointments to assess the situation and forge a new plan. The sudden allergic reaction had developed as a side effect of the toxic medicines.

I tried every remedy I could—detoxifying baths, burn gels, natural treatments, and cleansing foods—to strategically remove the toxins from my body. I wanted to get rid of every trace of the drugs I had just subjected myself to, unable to be assured that anything was helpful or working.

My hair steadily came out with every stroke of a hairbrush. Broad patches thinned and exposed my pale scalp. I felt looming pressure to quickly cut it off to make the loss feel less out of control.

I learned that since every fast-growing cell in my body had just been killed, my fingernails, surprisingly, might begin to peel off. I pulled at them cautiously to test their strength but detected no change.

I do not remember ending the dose, walking out of the hospital, or arriving back home on chemo day. I only recall the love necessary to manage the experience. I can still see the faces of the nurses and of the friends I made in the chairs around me, and I recall relying on my husband, who picked up all the slack on a day when there was a great deal of it.

Not everyone has the opportunity or resources to ask what chemotherapy is like. The experience was challenging to walk through and to write out, and I imagine it is challenging to read about.

RADIATION

Locker number five. I chose it daily, mindlessly making something familiar for myself in this unfamiliar place. Gown up, take everything off from the waist up, put my stuff in the cubbyhole, and swipe the patient ID card I had been assigned. Locker number five was the only thing I could intentionally claim as mine in this scenario. Nothing was familiar or predictable. I hated the room, the clothes, the story, and this entire process.

The generic-looking ID card, secured to a stretchy coil bracelet around my wrist, contained only a black barcode and some numbers. When I put it on, I felt reduced to a statistic, a diagnosis, a number, and a case. I inserted it into a machine, and a weak, bald picture of me filled the screen. In it I looked pale and slight and not like myself at all. My expression was lifeless, and it was unlike my usual personality. It was a deflating mirror image of more of what this process had taken away. I was not generic or a number. I was not usually sick or bald-headed. The card did not depict my life or who I was. I had not found myself in that place by choice.

Sitting here scarcely dressed in this waiting room, I felt I had done my part. The team had been alerted that I was ready, although mentally I was not. I waited somberly for the radiology nurse to retrieve me. I resumed the blank stare that had been interrupted from the day before. I was cold, uncomfortable, and feeling less than and diminished in the faded wraparound gown.

Whew. Same routine every day. The radiation would last for six and a half weeks, I had been informed. During the last week, they would increase my dose in a final effort to kill any resistant cancer-growing cells. Only now do I realize what was missing from that statement: an honest discussion about the effects that radiation would have on my body and the question "Would you like to have radiation?"

Why? Why was this happening? How did I get here? So much was occurring and moving through this season quickly, yet every day dragged on, heavy with content. My breast was sore, and my skin was blistered and raw. I had intense burns, and hours after the radiation treatments were over, the heat came off my body as the burns surfaced. It felt so wrong to subject such sensitive tissue to this treatment day after day on purpose. Radiation humiliates, stings, and damages deep within. If I had not felt sick before, I did now.

I met two different oncology patients, each named Lisa, in this room. The first Lisa entered the room confidently and launched into a casual conversation as if it were the norm to be there. She was friendly, articulate and matter-of-fact as she shared. She had an extreme story, and to listen to her explain it, one would think she could have had her own reality show.

She relayed that her breast cancer had been diagnosed in such an unusual way, through a bone being fractured in her leg. Unexpectedly, after never having been sick, she was suddenly in the middle of a gripping cancer tale that she did not appear dismantled by.

She was slightly entertaining, clearly doctor-shopping, and looking for answers beyond what she was being told. I was not there. As she talked, I tried to grasp her story but could not even grasp my own. She was a strong fighter. I wondered what I would be like when I tumbled out of this unpredictable and demanding season.

The second Lisa was more complicated for me to understand. An eclectic mix of anger and loss of reality, she described her experience of challenging doctors, second opinions, and information she learned from Web searches. She was confrontational and pushy and felt the need to fight off the slightest hint of sympathy. She also took her wig off freely to expose a naked scalp and did not give it a second thought or care.

I was still figuring out how I felt about all this. I could not imagine a time when I would ever be able to say any of those things or openly take my wig off. Watching her and considering this approach, I did not think it was a pattern I could follow. I sat in that room day after day, feeling as if I had no handle on any part of this illness. I found relief in hiding my naked scalp, trying to take part in my regular life, and keeping my concerns and fears locked away and cautiously hidden.

I have five tattoos from my experience with radiation. My tattoos are noticeable dark ink spots that I was told were necessary to mark the coordinates on my breast for the radiation treatments. That seems trivial, except I was against getting a tattoo on my body. My son had always talked about and wanted a tattoo. I always said, "Don't. You will regret it." I was receiving tattoos at the very moment I was learning that I was getting them. I was also told not to worry, that they would fade and were not permanent. I had no warning; there was no discussion; and I was given no other choice. Nobody asked me if putting a tattoo on my body was OK. I regret these tattoos.

Had I been asked, I may have chosen to agree to have them,

but in a season where I felt that I had been given no options, one more permanent choice had been taken away. I added getting tattoos to the information overload already in my head that night. Years later, I still have my five tattoos. There is no sign of fading, and they are as fresh as they were the day they were placed. They appear to be very permanent.

If not for the wonderfully encouraging and kind team of nurses who led me down the long winding hall daily to the mighty machine, learned about my life, and always met me with a friendly greeting, I would not have made it through or chosen to show up. They remembered who I was, something about me, and my story every single day. They were invested in me and distracted me with the inside scoop on the best restaurants they frequented near the hospital and other purposefully mindless topics. In hindsight, I imagine they knew I would like to walk away every time. It would not have taken much for me to find a reason not to show up.

Many times, I thought about skipping those appointments. I had a headful of legitimate excuses that I could justify and use. How much easier my day would be without the draining interruption of radiation: driving to the hospital, navigating the weak faces and the wheelchairs, and making my way to the elevator to get to the third floor, where I walked past the empty salon with the outdated wigs in the window, beyond the daunting infusion center, and through the doors to the oncology radiation waiting area.

I would be directed to lie down on the cold steel table in the position rehearsed the day before. With my gown open, the radiation tech would manipulate my breast tissue to line it up with the machine, check the coordinates, evacuate the room, and tell me to hold still from beyond the wall.

These people became my trusted friends. I instantly relied on them to protect my life. I had to. I knew they were waiting for me in the other room and would return after they pushed the button and gave the all clear. If I had nothing else, I would have confidence in their skillfulness and care. They were overseeing a wave of radiation that, in too high a dose, had the ability to end an unsuspecting patient's life.

There were nature graphics on the ceiling meant to distract. An image of cherry trees in blossom that were otherwise out of place in a sterile procedure room. These never distracted me enough to take my mind off what was happening. This was hard and unsettling. It was happening faster than I could think it through, and the reality of why I was there was unnerving. That daily invisible zap of radiation drained every bit of my energy in a single moment as I wondered what else it was doing that I could not see.

During one of those hallway conversations, one of the nurses asked me how I was managing a full-time job. I told her that I was doing OK but was very tired every day when I returned to work. She pressed the issue and asked how my job was treating me. I said that they allowed me to have an extra-long lunch and were understanding and that I was appreciative for that. I had time to get to the hospital each day, complete the treatment, pick up food, and return to my desk.

This appointment always took longer than a typical lunch break would ever allow for. The nurse went on to explain that she had patients who lost their jobs because the radiation caused so much exhaustion and, as a result, work productivity declined. Until then, I had not considered that the loss of a job could be one more toll cancer could unexpectedly take on my life.

I was grateful for my nurses and for this experience as I moved on, aware that the outcome could have been quite different. Later, when radiation was behind me, I learned of a patient in another clinic who had died from having mistakenly been given too high a radiation dose. Not that it would have helped me, but had I known all the dangers at every appointment, I may have sat in that waiting room and thoughtfully considered what was happening instead of donning my vacant stare.

At my last appointment, the small team gathered in the room and congratulated me with a certificate of completion to honor my last dose. It was unexpected and bittersweet. They had become part of my journey, and I would fondly miss them. Each one had written something so thoughtful and personal that I saved it. There were hugs and genuine tears as I saw the human compassion that was always there beyond their professionalism. I had now graduated, and they celebrated with me. Years later, I still remember the conversations, recall those vivid pictures, and have those fond memories locked in my mind.

Moving forward, doctors would often ask me, "When was your last radiation?" I have a reference that I can easily remember, Good Friday. Jesus died on Good Friday. My cells were dead, and my breast was burned by Good Friday. By Friday, I suspected the tattoos were permanent. By Friday, I was on to the next phase of treatment with new sores and blisters that would continue surfacing over the next several weeks. *This chapter is over. Never again,* I said to myself. I made it to Friday.

OVERWHELMED

I was there in that radiologist's office because I had cancer. I never planned for or expected cancer. Before this journey, I never knew the exact role of a radiology oncologist. I waited in this room for them to tell me whether I was healing well or not. I had learned to smile cautiously, exchange pleasantries, and walk through the process, but that did not mean I was not derailed by this experience and struggling through every step. I had been to this office too many times over the past several weeks and was continuously reminded of how many more appointments were still ahead.

There was a sign propped up on the counter near the sink in the otherwise sterile office, and I read it in dismay. "Overwhelmed? We can help," it said. The bare office held only basic medical equipment for gathering patient vitals. The walls were pale gray-blue, drab, and cold, with no pictures to distract my attention. There was nothing else to look at, so the sign stood out significantly. I anxiously sat on the edge of the elevated exam table feeling like nothing but a shell around a disease and waiting for the door to open and the monotonous exchange to begin once again.

Like a newborn, I was scheduled to return there in three weeks, six weeks, three months, etc. I heard the doctor name the appointments out five years, and I thought, *Five years? I will not be able to leave this behind me for five years? That is overwhelming. Irony. Yes, I am overwhelmed!* It is not what I say, but if you could see past my minimal responses and the blank expression on my face and hear my thoughts, you would be assured that yes, I was entirely overwhelmed.

I did not want to be there. I did not like this process, and I did not like what I had learned this treatment would now do to my body long term. This was never made clear to me. During each visit, I heard a bit more about the side effects, one by one, as I brought my concerning symptoms to the doctor's attention. It felt as though the accurate picture had been deceptively held back, and I was not a fan of this method, which felt like an unfair guessing game. I was secretly hoping this all would end just as mysteriously as it started. Name one part of this that was not overwhelming!

The radiology oncologist and I exchange casual greetings, and I even agree when he remembers the wrong sex of my children. Correcting him was pointless and insignificant compared to why I was here. No part of me wanted to engage in a long-term relationship with this doctor. I had carefully self-protected and guarded against any more of my identity being stolen in this situation. I decided at the very moment that I chose not to correct him that he was not part of my important team. He had no idea who I really was or how this season was affecting me.

This journey started when I was forty-nine years old, comfortable with myself, content with life, and working at the usual challenges. My children ranged in age from twelve to twenty years at the time of my diagnosis. I had a full-time career as an administrator for a professional law enforcement organization and believed in the people I worked for and my position.

I loved to bake, laugh, paint, and decorate. I enjoyed planning family vacations and valued my time on any beach. I was personable and genuinely enjoyed helping people. I was a believer who was passionate about my faith. My life was predictable. I felt whole. That was who I was, and it did not include anything about cancer or why I was sitting on this exam table feeling unknown and subtracted from.

I located the tissue box next to the sign. More irony. This was not a place I wanted to be when I processed how overwhelmed I felt. If I were to share my feelings, I would be offered a prescription, warned again about depression, and had references made to all the obvious things that I already knew I should be doing: get more rest, exercise, try not to worry, blah blah blah. I would have loved to rest, but I had forgotten what that was in this season. I slept little, and most of it was not restful. Exercise would have been great, but I had stitches that were still dissolving, swelling, pain, and new hurdles I had never had before. I struggled to manage daily life and could not see a time when it would change. There was a lot to think through, consider, and reflect on. This daily exhaustion from subjecting my body to radiation was completely consuming, and there was no room to add anything else. I had listened. I knew all too well this routine.

I discreetly blotted three more tears than I had planned to let out and left. I was not depressed; I was only tired, and there was nobody there to explain this to. And even if I did explain it, it would never matter. I was in the middle of a solo walk, and there was no other choice before me but to keep to the schedule and keep on going.

After my radiation appointment, I would return to my job at my empty office and keep my eyes open as I watched the clock slowly crawl through the afternoon to half past four. My office remained unusually quiet with little requirement on my part over those several weeks of appointments. In hindsight, I realized the gift of space my employers gave me, purposely and mercifully. To this day, I think fondly and remain grateful that I worked for a compassionate group of people who valued me and respected me enough to give me the space I needed to manage the season and all it included.

When I first had to tell my employers, a mostly male-dominated office, that I had breast cancer, they were solemn, thoughtful, accommodating, and empathetic. In very few carefully chosen words, I was told they had decided that I would never run out of sick time. Nevertheless, I felt guilty for entertaining the idea of leaving work unfinished, taking time off, or admitting that I needed it. Not that this would not have been understood and respected, but I pushed myself and did not allow the relief my body needed during this time.

What little I could manage while having cancer was focused on my trying to control how far it could push me and guarding what I would not let it take away. While everything foreign was happening, I poured my efforts into not appearing weak and fought off even the slightest idea that I was not able to keep up with everything that I had been able to do before.

It was increasingly difficult day after day to focus on my computer screen and keep my head lifted at my desk. There were days when I resisted nodding my head multiple times to keep from falling asleep. Radiation, although I did not understand all it was doing inside my body, was exhaustingly consuming beyond anything I had ever experienced.

And so it went that I continued to have several days of radiation, meet with the radiology oncologist, have several more days of radiation, and so on. I dragged myself through the routine in and out of every appointment and schedule. I never understood those brief meetings to be anything other than a formality. When I shared my concern about the deepening blisters and the pain and showed the doctor the severe burns, it was nothing surprising or new that he had not seen before. There was little he had to offer in terms of remedy or remark. There was no discussion about how to navigate my life with these new challenges or what I could expect next.

I remained distanced, formal, and emotionless throughout these repetitive appointments, all the way to the end. These meetings gave me no more helpful information than I already had, and besides, that doctor was not in the room when the button was pushed, nor was he part of our important hallway connections.

Not knowing where this illness would take me, I kept to my regular schedule, working full time, coffee cup in hand. If I could speak to my younger self after what I have learned now, I would give permission to scale back and take some personal time; offering the reminder that it is OK to rest. I am not defined by what I can accomplish or how much I could do. I was created to care for people, and I should have made it a priority to do that for myself.

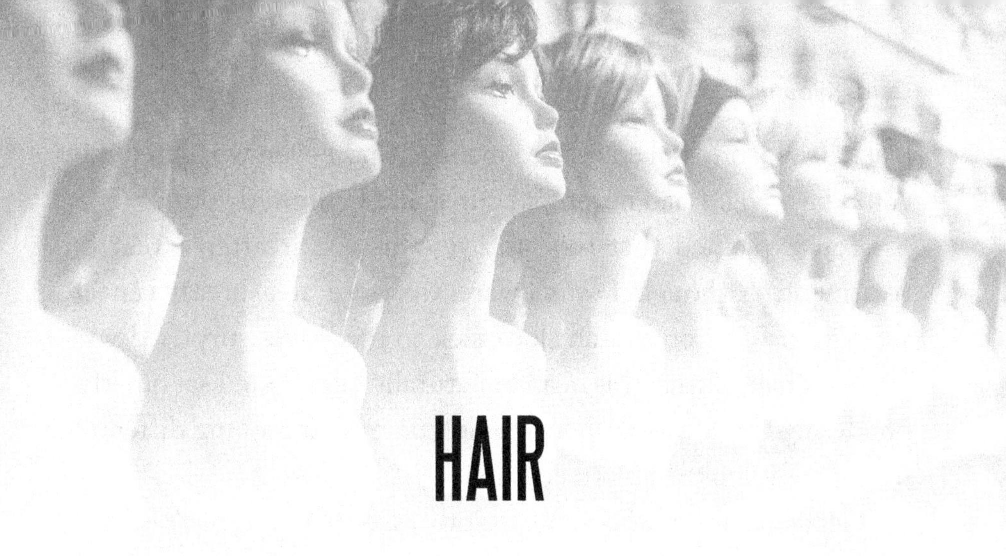

HAIR

I had been walking through the treatments for about six months and trying to get up the courage to attend one of the breast cancer support groups. The hosting organization was near my work, and the women I had met were understanding and supportive, offering financial and emotional resources. When they handed me their calendar and encouraged me to attend, I felt obligated to try a meeting at least once. Breast cancer is a popular form of this disease, so tangible resources like the ones this organization deliver are easily found and more widely available.

I walked into the large, open conference room, past the plate of packaged cookies and stale-smelling coffee. The space was filled with women sitting at long empty tables. So much conversation was being exchanged that I felt as if I was the only one with no connection. It was not what I expected, although I had no idea what to expect. I sat down next to you because you looked friendly and appeared to be alone. I finally got the courage to tell you your hair was cute, and you mildly scoffed at my remark, saying you did not like it.

Your quick, definitive answer took me off guard, and I could give no reply. Your short, tight curls were pushed back by a thick black headband, looked easy to manage, and I even wondered if it could be a wig. I had never had curls, and I admired yours.

You explained that this was your new hair after a year of treatment. Although I was aware we were at a breast cancer support group, you did not look sick to me. I was surprised you were not happy with this head of naturally curly hair. I sat quietly, pondering the idea that hair would come back looking different from how it looked before chemo.

I glanced around the room, quietly assessing everyone's hair. *Is it real? Have they also lost their hair? Is it a battle for them too?* My eyes wandered around the room as I wondered if I was the only one battling such thoughts. I had no idea if these were the game faces of every woman in here and if they too struggled with the things I struggled with.

I hid a bald scalp under this thick wig that you may not have known was not my natural hair. I never offered that information because I was ashamed and embarrassed sitting there that I did not have anything underneath it. It seemed deceptive, but I had kept myself so busy in that season that I barely had the space to think about how that made me feel.

I can remember nothing else about that day. Every thought was directed toward hair, how overwhelming the loss felt, and what to do to manage the information I had just learned. My straight, medium-brown hair was a little past my shoulders when I was diagnosed. The time I had been given to get it cut off was running out, and I knew it had to be done soon. I had heard stories of brave women who planned an appointment to get a short new hairstyle in a salon surrounded by friends. I had never been particularly good at masking my feelings or finding any part of this situation I could approach lightheartedly and publicly.

I devised my own plan, one that I could handle privately. My husband agreed to cut my hair short at home, and then I would start wearing the wig I had purchased while I waited for the rest of it to fall out. I was not ready, but there would never be a time when I would be. We agreed on the day to do it, and when the evening came, there was no more time left for me to stall. I had been mindlessly watching TV, letting the hours pass and putting the task off for as long as possible.

Finally, I stood up and announced, "Let's do it now." My husband was surprised and questioned my timing, but that was how I tended to manage a challenge I dreaded. I was at a loss now for much of a conversation or explanation. I went to the mirror, gathered my hair in a ponytail, and sat on our small bathroom rug. My son, who was home from college, held up my ponytail, and with some noticeable hesitation, my husband took the scissors and, with one cut, cautiously snipped it off. I could only imagine their faces when it was done and it was cut off. I was glad I could not see their expressions. I assume they were regretful or apologetic, but neither said a word. There was no conversation. Both would have done anything to help that I asked them to do. I now cannot imagine doing the same thing for someone else. In hindsight, it was a sad milestone to have to share.

Two weeks after chemotherapy, just as I had been warned by my doctor, my hair began to fall out. It was unstoppable, painful, traumatic, and still surprising despite the warnings. Right on schedule, it fell out steadily and quickly. Much to my surprise, I learned that losing one's hair hurts. My balding head began to feel burned and raw, and lying down on a pillow was overwhelmingly painful. I wrapped fluffy fabric around my head to cushion the pain of sleeping at night. It took several uncomfortable days to fall completely out. As it did so, I lost my identity as I no longer recognized the person I saw looking back in the mirror.

No hat exists that feels comforting or natural on a suddenly bald scalp. Bald feels cold, itchy, vulnerable, and uncomfortable. At home, I typically wore a cotton hat and favored it over the itchy wig that now smelled like the coconut oil I used to condition it. I had some beautiful scarves but needed to improve at fashioning a head wrap from a scarf. I tried it once, and without warning it slipped off my naked scalp in public. I went through sheer panic to quickly gather the slick fabric again, knot it, and get it back on my head without drawing any attention. The wig became my go-to for easy coverage and the best chance I had of hiding this sickness, which I was now adamant about doing.

Hair is familiar, identifying, predictable, and always yours. My focus was understandably on the hair on my head until, one day, I discovered that my eyebrows were mostly gone, and I had only three eyelashes left on one eye. I remember having learned that people typically have around a hundred eyelashes on each eye. It was unnerving to notice such a small enough number to be able to count them.

I had not considered the effect that losing my eyelashes, eyebrows, or body hair would have until it happened. It was all just suddenly gone as if it had never been there, with no notice or sign that any of it would ever return. I was surprisingly hairless for months, with no guarantee any of it would come back.

Later, when my eyelashes started to grow back, it was just as remarkable as initially losing them was. Slowly, they came in, short and thin; maybe that was all they would ever be. Then they became full, normal, almost surprising—the outcome as peculiar as the onset of the loss.

With eight months of slow hair growth, I had at best what I called a mismanaged boy haircut that I sometimes bothered to put a headband in. I mostly left it untouched as I did not want to show my approval or appreciation for this unwelcome result.

My thickening baby-soft hair was one shade darker, curly, and short for the first time ever. I was not a fan at all. I had yet to blow-dry, style, or work with my new head of hair. I respected what it took to grow, as irrational as it sounds, and I did not want to challenge it to fall out again.

I would walk by a mirror, catch a glimpse, and think, *I am not me. Who is that?* Then I would remember, and the thought quickly came, *This is my new normal, the one I was warned about. I look like this now, and I cannot do much to change it.* I noticed any hair loss now and wondered if it was happening all over again. I noted any eyelash that fell out and hoped these new ones would stay.

Hair is the outward sign of an inward process. It is how we describe ourselves and differentiate ourselves one from one another. It also can depict our sense of style, our confidence, and our personality. I combed back, ignored, refused to focus on, and avoided dealing with my new hair at all costs.

I read somewhere that a cancer patient had struggled to explain to a hairdresser why all her hair was the same length. It remained unthinkable for me to imagine going back to a salon to navigate any type of conversation. It took time for me to gain the courage to ask a professional how to care for this new hair, allowing some of it to be cut off and confidently believing it would grow again. Because of that, I waited a year from the day my radiation had ended to take this step and enter a hair salon again.

I hesitantly made the appointment and walked in. I could tell by the perplexed look on the stylist's face that she had forgotten who I was, but there was something familiar she recalled about me. It had been a long time, and I did not look the same as she must have remembered.

Right away, before she asked too many questions or noticed my hair was all one length, I spilled out an abbreviated version of my story in one long breath. She listened intently but showed little reaction to my words, then graciously led me past the other customers and stylists to her station in the back.

Others could hear our conversation in the busy salon, and she was considerate with every word. I felt overwhelmed and anxious and was worried I might start to cry uncontrollably. The stylist's mom had died of breast cancer, she explained. Not exactly what I wanted to hear at the time. She had tended to her hair care and expressed that she understood my challenges.

She went on to wash and cut my hair as she carefully encouraged and reassured me through every step. I could tell from her reserved exchanges that she was also struggling to visit her own painful memories.

I got a brand-new short haircut that I did not like that day. I pretended to like it but could not wait to get out of that chair, pay my bill, and leave. Nothing about being in that place would have made any of it better. Feeling powerless, I had no private option to manage what was left of my former head of hair.

I made it through that appointment and thanked her. I was grateful to have a place that felt familiar on a day filled with so much apprehension. As I said goodbye, she unexpectedly hugged me. I will never forget the bond we shared after struggling through that first together, but I hope that she understands why I will never come back to sit in her chair.

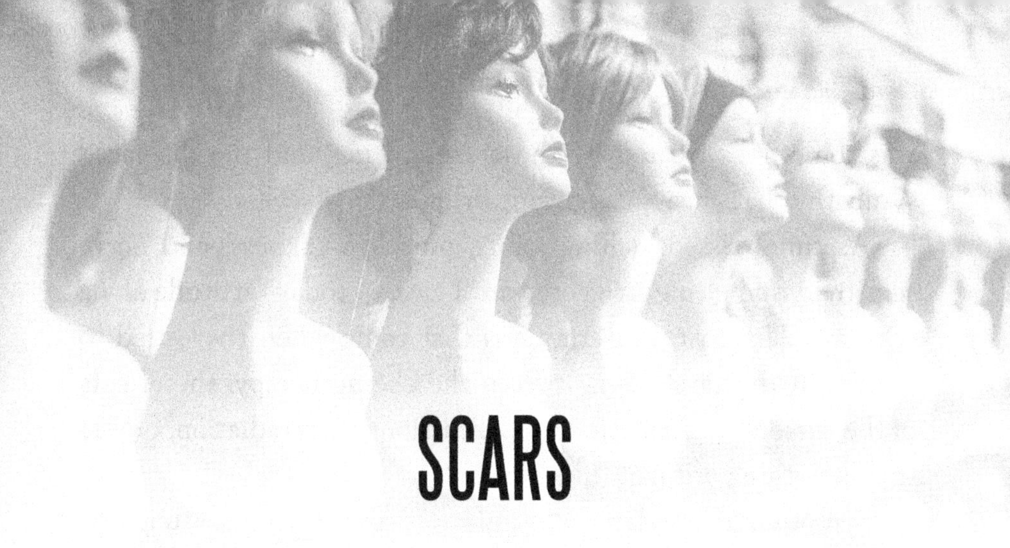

SCARS

My scars became constant reminders of the apparent attack. They are the gash line in my armpit used to remove the lymph nodes that I did not know were going to be taken out that day; the long, straight line on my breast where the tumor was cut out and the staples were now inserted; and the noticeable thick concave scar forever left near my collarbone, which is oddly shaped and appears uneven and crudely cut.

For months, the site was where the plastic port marked the opening to my body, allowing the chemo drugs to flow straight to my heart. When the chemo port was removed, it was learned that I had been allergic to its materials and had been fighting its presence in my body. Because my body rejected the port, the mark is jagged, the area swollen and tender, and the wound complex. After a series of painful steroid shots directly into the tissue, the irregular scarred result was the best it would ever be.

There are also hidden scars that cannot be seen. I have heard them described when I have listened to myself retell my story as the years have passed. They are the moments of unexpected, unfair despair I saw my children endure; the weariness in my husband's eyes as he worked not to miss anything; the new fragile way I was sometimes treated by those around me; and the displaced sympathy that always caught me off guard.

As time passed, aching joints, muscle weakness, and nerve sensitivity sometimes triggered an "I give up today" attitude along with a roller coaster of emotions that came when I wrestled to figure out the cause. Was it from the chemotherapy, the effects of the current medication, or repercussions from radiation, or was this something ordinary like a virus?

Symptoms marked my path and lasted for years in the aftermath of the medicines, treatments, and therapies. With the progression of age, it became impossible to separate the side effects of cancer treatments from the natural ailments of growing older. A new normalcy in my life emerged that became defined by a forced focus on navigating health challenges.

My husband and I stepped out of our usual routine for a short, much-needed vacation, our first since this medical journey had begun a little more than a year before. Having time to relax and space to think meant dealing with those feelings I had been stuffing and doing my best to silence and avoid.

We were in the resort pool, and he casually but pointedly asked how I was doing. I knew what he was inquiring about, but my entire body stiffened as I began to panic. It was part of a conversation I had hoped not to bring along with me. We had been married for a decade at this point. He is thoughtful and compassionate and had been with me through every step of this, and I had not been able to hide much.

I tried to give a superficial, casual answer, but I was struggling at the moment. He cares, and I have always been able to express my best and worst thoughts to him. There were so many pieces of it that I wanted to talk through, but not when I felt overwhelmed. When I could no longer hold the tears in, I bobbed underwater and returned to the surface with an entirely wet face. I chose not to share it with him this time. I hid from him the fact that there were tears in the mix, and he had no idea that anything was haunting me at that moment.

I hid my feelings because I did not want to be comforted and did not wish to realize I needed to be. It already had taken so much to convince myself to search for and wear a bathing suit that evened out the new lumps and drew enough attention away from the apparent scars. At this point, that was all I could see in the mirror. The overall picture was bleak. There was no indication it would change, and I could not imagine dumping all that on my husband in the middle of this pool.

I did not know what cancer should look or feel like. I was navigating this the best way I could figure out moment by moment. Everyone has something they struggle with. I stand in line behind a stranger in the grocery store, and I am unaware of the pain they have suffered from losing their baby. I am oblivious when the barista makes my custom cup of coffee that he is battling with the incredible loss of his marriage. When my mechanic services my car, I am unmindful of the fact that his child was in a terrible life-altering accident and that he has no other means but to be here to pay those bills.

We all have trials, wounds, scars, and victories. Life can be as challenging as it is rewarding and as lonely as it is comforting. I do not try to compare my trouble to that of others. Mine is all I know, and I feel obligated to share mine if it could help with someone else's.

I sometimes pictured myself flinging my wig in the air as my situation spun out of control, but nothing was lighthearted about any of this. Cancer felt the opposite of that. It was taxing as we awaited the next appointment, the subsequent treatment, and the next plan. Also, cancer is not just cancer. Cancer is a winding trail that comes with unknown baggage in the form of complex therapies that affect the body in negative unforeseen ways.

With the presence of a cancer diagnosis, my doctors were alerted to watch for more potential risks and side effects. I witnessed several of these developments when sleeplessness, heart irregularities, hormone issues, and questionable scan results were all detected. Cancer opened the door for new diagnostics, with many more questions and concerns that came along with them, as every medical professional had a heightened concern about my history.

As a result of that in-depth monitoring, I endured multiple medical investigations, including a monitored sleep study with electrodes glued to my head, and multiple scans to identify new masses to rule out additional cancers. And my heart suddenly became the focus of specialists and around-the-clock monitoring when an unusual heart rhythm emerged in the aftermath of chemotherapy. A few years later, I was sent to the hospital after a routine physical to assess a slight elevation in numbers indicating the possibility of a blood clot in my lungs.

I scheduled my first annual "scared-a-gram" (mammogram) and held my breath. Once again, I put all my belongings in an empty locker and sat on the bench in the back room waiting area. Wrapped in a thin smock and feeling subjected, I anxiously anticipated my flesh being manipulated and situated on the cold machine. I played all the scenarios in my head while waiting there. How would I tell my husband that they had called me back again? How soon would I need to, if there was a better way, and what were any or all my choices this time? I remained braced for the worst on the inside, and I was not sure if that would ever change.

Thankfully, this time, I had a thoughtful technician who asked me if I would like to see my results instead of ignoring the history in the chart she had just been given. She took me over to her computer and showed me the comparison on the screen of my past three films, including the cancer mass. It was the first time I saw what had caused all the trouble. The cloudy mass on the X-ray film was distinct and very noticeable. The cancer did not hide. It was clear, distinctive and stood out from everything else around it.

I looked at the comparison for the first time, and something about it was helpful and settling for me. I no longer had to wonder what it looked like; was it easily hidden, able to have been missed? I had seen the cancer mass, and it appeared noticeable, obvious, and I suspect, identifiable to a professional trained eye.

LONELY

You stood in front of me alone, in the line to the women's room, and I was very distracted by your turban. I saw you self-consciously pull at it, ensuring it was touching your ear and hiding every part of your naked head. It was thin, and your smooth scalp still peeked through.

There were so many things I wanted to say to you, but we had never met. I noticed the orange tinge on your skin and could surmise your chemo treatments were current. I tried to meet your eyes and look for an opening, anything to connect. I did not want to stare, so I hoped you would look up and acknowledge me. Undeniably, you must have felt my eyes fixed on you. I would have taken any indication as an invitation that it was OK to start a conversation.

Maybe I could help. Maybe I knew. After all, somehow, we were involuntary members of the same club. My treatments were over, but I was curious to learn how you found out. Perhaps it could continue to help me with the aftermath of my thoughts and questions. Maybe we had the same story, and I could help you feel that this walk was not so lonely.

I followed you out the door, a few steps behind, searching for any appropriate words to call to your back as you got away. I missed my chance and was filled with regret because I remembered. Although I hid under my wig for a long time and refused to wear the pink slogans, I was lonely and longed for connections. Ugh! I missed my chance with you and am unsure which of us needed the connection more.

As my last radiation treatment was approaching, I was invited to join a women's cancer wellness group in our small community. I do not remember how they found me or how I found them, but I was grateful for the new connection. It was the kind of practical resource I had desperately needed and had been unsure if such a thing existed. This first year of managing the cancer diagnosis had left me feeling isolated, singled out, and desperate for like-minded friends who could effortlessly relate.

Around the table sat five other women of various ages. Each was afflicted with some form of cancer in various stages of recovery, understanding, and coping. We shared, connected, and empathized with one another. They were some of the most honest and pain-filled conversations I have ever been present for. These women had become my support, a network of understanders and been-theres who could relate to what I felt and experienced. They each had a family, a story, and an ongoing battle.

The facilitator, having had a mother who survived breast cancer, posed the question to each of us, "What is the hardest part of this journey?" The woman next to me answered at once: "Loneliness." Cancer is lonely. It isolates, traps, and detaches, leaving an individual with a new mindset, a new way of life, and a new thought process even before he or she realizes that it is happening. At best, do-gooders and well-wishers touch on the problem for a moment or during a conversation, but then it is back to the isolated walk nobody can fully understand or do in a cancer patient's place.

"My biggest fear is that it will come back again." I heard her say those words, and I was not far enough along in this process to have realized that thought on my own. She was close to my age and had described a family with children like mine. There was desperation in her voice, and she blinked back tears as she told of her battle.

Cancer is a looming enemy. Those who have never grappled with the idea of cancer cells multiplying within their bodies have not experienced the suffocating weight of having brought desperation to those they were meant to care for and protect.

Everyone around the table had a painful story with different details. They had lost friends who did not know what to say, male family members who walked away any time the word *breast* was mentioned, and relationships that took an adverse turn in the face of hardship.

I was still working to sort through my own story. I had never thought of my cancer coming back. But sitting here listening to this woman and understanding how she arrived honestly at this concern, I now shared her biggest fear.

One woman described that she felt utterly abandoned by her friends. They were a close small group who planned something together every week. After a few times of having to say she could not be there, they had stopped asking. She could no longer take part in the same activities as she had before the cancer, so she was now left out.

I wished I could speak to those friends and tell them that now more than ever, they should have encircled her, discovered some new plans she could be a part of, and at least for now, kept her in the middle and held tight to her because she was scared. Loneliness would be the worst thing and one more thing she could not bear, especially right now.

Each story came with tears—bottled up, labeled, and stored,

but still very raw. No sentiments or conclusions could be offered. There were no appropriate "look on the bright side" or "try harder" approaches. We had no expectation other than to listen and genuinely empathize with one another because we understood. It was simply about sharing and letting out what had been weighty and too overwhelming to keep quiet and hidden.

Another woman shared that every time her doctor explained reasonable limits that he could foresee in her near future, her husband told her that those things would not happen. The problem arose after every doctor appointment. She grew increasingly frustrated. In his delusion, optimism, or plain denial, her husband just did not seem to be listening. Instead of counting on his support to help her through what was inevitably to come, she had to convince him of her needs and train him to accept her new norm and help her through it.

I shared a card with the group that I had received from a friend shortly after my diagnosis. On the front was a dinosaur alone on an island watching Noah and his ark sail away from him. The slogan was "Oh no, was that today?" And on the inside, it read, "Some days are just like that." I smiled when I opened it and hung it somewhere I could see it often. She understood. Cancer felt completely out of control; it just happened to me, and there were no fitting thoughts that could be expressed. "I am sorry this happened to you" was a very appropriate—and the only—sentiment necessary to express.

The support group disbanded—something about schedules and prior commitments. To know it was there meant so much to me that I could not bring myself to respond to the casual text as each party dropped out. The group had been canceled by default. Cancer does not wait to show up until it is scheduled. It interrupts, bulldozes, flattens, contaminates, and then changes everything in its path. It is interruptive, inconvenient, and dismantling. It is a new filter nobody wants. It builds up, and when the feelings that accompany it can no longer be stuffed in, they surface.

In honor of those women who shared their stories, I created a list of ways to help someone experiencing cancer. I want to share them with you on behalf of any person who needs you to know what they are:

- ✓ Do not overthink the should-I's. Be the one to send the card or flowers, drop off the meal, or make the phone call.
- ✓ Never let someone you care about go to chemotherapy alone.
- ✓ Ask, "How are you feeling?"; "What can I do?"; "How can I help?" Then keep asking.
- ✓ Assume it is more challenging than you know, and be the best friend/sibling/spouse you can be.
- ✓ Listen more than you advise.
- ✓ Be a safe person with whom to share, cry, despair, or triumph.
- ✓ Make contact through phone calls, cards, hugs, and prayers. Contact is critical.
- ✓ Know that everyone needs help. Shop, mow, clean, give, and find a way to help compensate for what is difficult, impossible, or forgotten in the lives of those struggling.
- ✓ Provide an opportunity for the person to talk and process things honestly without judgment.
- ✓ Understand that cancer is expensive, time-consuming, frustrating, and exhausting.
- ✓ Adjust to the changes, the information, and the emotions. Cancer is demanding and messy for everyone.

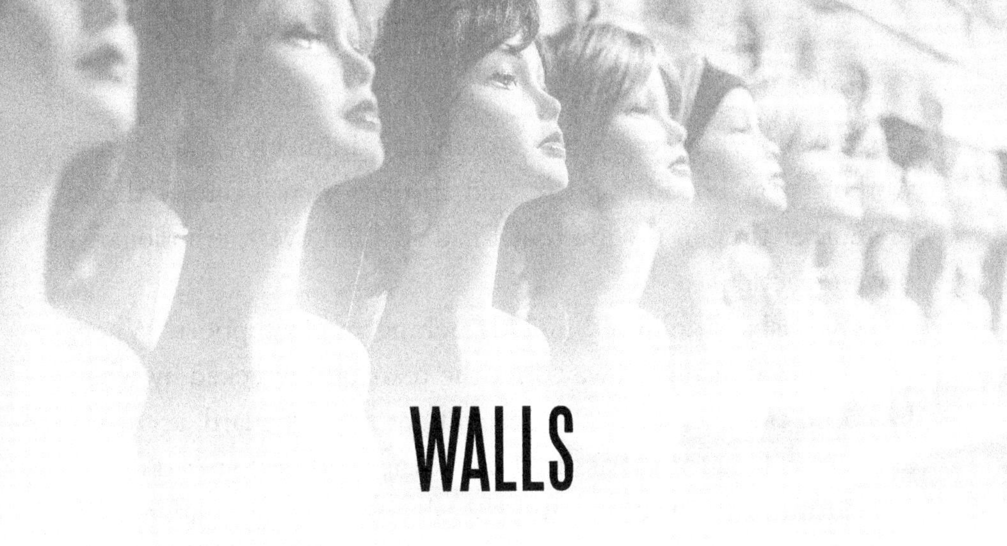

WALLS

We were at a Bible study at church when the leader recklessly stated that cancer purposely happened to some families, suggesting that it was something I had deserved. The air suddenly felt as though it were filled with blame. There were only fourteen people in the room, and although it should have felt safe, the walls suddenly closed in on me. It was as if there was not enough oxygen or space. I panicked. My guard was down. I had been sitting there, encouraged by the content, so it was the last thing I expected to hear.

It had been a little more than a year since my treatments had ended, and I was adjusting to its aftereffects and some of the new normal in my life. I was apprehensive about sharing my fight with cancer, remaining guarded as I sorted privately through my own questions and feelings. I kept my own unrealistic thoughts of self-blame for having grown this tumor buried inside, to protect myself.

Cancer felt raw, personal, and unresolved. There was no history, no curse, and no way I could have seen it coming. It was something that happened to me, but I still wrestled with the responsibility for its presence and development.

Sitting beside me, my husband had heard the same unfair, inaccurate account and must have understood how it made me feel. He also appeared restless and anxious as the conversation progressed. Without any verbal exchange, I quickly gathered my workbook, grabbed my purse, and abruptly fled. I cannot think of another time in my life that I had such an overt, emotionally driven reaction.

My husband followed quickly behind me in support. When we got a safe distance away, I let the tears out, wrecked by what had been carelessly said. I felt caught entirely off guard, accused, and angry. He gently reassured me of the truth as I vowed never to return to that class. It is unbelievable how we can understand the facts and simultaneously be vulnerable to lies.

We live in a world with pollutants and toxins and excellent diagnostic equipment. We are an innovative, proactive society medically responsible for our bodies. With better diagnostics and screenings, sometimes cancer is detected. When it is, wherever it is, one needs to believe there is no fault to be assigned. Sad things happen, as do good things, every day across the world. Without faith, we would think there is no purpose for these trials or triumphs. Without faith, I would not have had a place to find the strength to face my struggles and be grateful for my victories. There would be no separation between good and evil and no way to distinguish the wins when they happened. Without walking through my difficulties, I could not encourage anyone else through theirs.

I braced myself two weeks later with a newfound determination to face the same group with the truth. I sat silently without making eye contact, fully absorbed in the strategic dialogue in my head. Quietly, I calculated how I might begin to unpack this and help everyone in the room hear me. I strained to push out the words carefully and methodically, trying against all odds to be steady and emotionless.

Nobody could have guessed it took everything I had to return and sit there to explain any of this. It also struck me as unfair that

I felt the responsibility to do so. But I could not leave any of the group members believing those lies spoken and labeled as truth in this room. Cancer steals enough, and because I personally had seen such a false and inaccurate account, I could not leave others deceived and believing those lies.

I began telling them all the highlights of what had happened to me as I moved quickly through my story, relating the main points and working to keep my voice steady. Reassuring the group that God would never punish us with sickness, I purposefully reminded them of who God is. "Please think more before you speak because you never know what someone else is going through and if they may take your words to heart as their truth. Cancer is filled with dark lies, and you do not have to believe any of them. Look at me. Let me tell you some good things about this difficult season.

"My kids had to look for, find, and adhere to God like never before. My eyes were opened to what love looks and acts like and how it never quits. And then there is trust. I trust like I never could before. I learned that I had to. We now live our lives appreciating each day. I work to be present every day and strive to look back with no regrets. I work to return love to those around me. I keep reaching for and finding a place to apply God's love. I work harder at everything, with purpose, to accomplish something worthy of whatever I put my hands to. I consider what I will be leaving behind one day and wonder if this day might be my last. Did I do enough? Cancer did try to steal, but I am only allowing it to leave behind the good that came from it."

At times, I paused and was at a loss for words, but when I was quiet, my husband picked up the cue and continued with more details. I was grateful for the boldness, tenacity, and space to speak the truth. Together, we impacted the narrative that day and changed the damage that had been deposited into the group.

PINK

I saw the giant pink swish on the office door while driving by on my lunch hour and just stopped in on a whim. The business was located in a strip mall that I had passed by many times before, but this was the first time I had noticed this place. I was searching for some new insight and a few more straightforward answers. I was sure that stumbling across this resource was a sign. For as long as cancer had been around, someone must have had better answers than the ones I had. I entered the door and noticed books and papers piled on desks and multiple whiteboards with lists. Hoping I had found the resources I desperately needed, I boldly interrupted a meeting between two women.

After a quick greeting, I was graciously ushered to a desk in the corner. As the questions swelled in my mind, I spilled out a condensed version of the story of my cancer journey. I was seeking information, nutrition help, and viable alternative options. The woman went from book to book, one source after another, really trying, but she found nothing—no alternate information could be located. My questions were too big, and no chapters anywhere contained streamlined or accessible answers. I needed definitive direction, confident help, and more effective resources.

I held back tears and composed myself as she stepped into

the walk-in closet to fish my size from a large open box of pink T-shirts. Although not a survivor, her mom had died of breast cancer years ago, she said. In her mother's honor, she worked to bring awareness and education to others facing the same daunting diagnosis.

Such a familiar story I learned over the years: volunteering in such an organization in a loved one's honor. She had been planning an annual fundraiser when I interrupted her, and she offered support in the form of an invitation to join those efforts.

It was my second pink cancer T-shirt, bright pink and with the same message, but the wording was a little different. The shirt had the word *survivor* on it. That did not fit who I thought I was. I did not feel like a survivor, whatever that was supposed to feel like. I felt like a depleted woman with three scars and five tattoos, none of which I was proud. I would not have chosen this battle, and I would not selflessly take it on again. I had done nothing heroic or unique. I showed up, kept to the schedule, and lived through it. I wished they would give me a shirt that said "Victim." I could justify wearing that.

I thanked the woman and hugged her as I parted. Not because of what she had handed me, but because I felt for the few minutes that she had listened that I was not alone in my situation or battle. I went back to wondering if there was any resource that could offer the help I was so desperately seeking.

I retold the story of that visit to a close friend who had known me for many years. I was sure she would understand and agree with how I felt. "Victim," I told her. "That is what I feel like I am."

She quickly contradicted me: "Victim is the last thing you are." Her answer perplexed me as I sorted through how I felt and responded to my circumstances and how others perceived my responses. I had been wrestling with the idea of feeling like a victim, but over time, I would eventually come to agree with her statement. She was right: I was not a victim.

I was not ready for a race, a walk, or even a small party. And I was not at the point where I could casually don a pink ribbon as if it were a part of my regular wardrobe. I also did not feel that I was part of any dynamic fighting team that had earned the right to proudly display one of these survivor shirts. I would start a pile somewhere of my pink T-shirts and save them for when this did not feel so raw and when pink could return to being my favorite color. I was not there just yet, which was OK because that day, it was the best I could do.

My first cancer T-shirt had been given to me by my husband only a few days after the diagnosis. He needed to do something, and this was where he focused his efforts. He felt compelled to buy himself and me matching T-shirts that said, "Fight like a girl." It was a sweet gesture, but they were still both in a pile and left unworn months later. I do not think either of us felt there was an appropriate day to wear these shirts confidently during that initial period of shock. There had not been a single time when I woke up and thought, *Today I am part of the united team. Let me find my shirt; I am ready to fight in this battle.* Instead, I would pick up where I had left off the day before. It was a mostly solitary, unnerving, unpredictable walk.

Unfortunately, even a well-thought-out gift could not change my prognosis. Instead, it was that someone who loved me would do anything and had to do something to share some of my burden. The real gift my husband gave to me was the reminder that this was happening to both of us and that I was not alone.

My favorite color is pink. I usually appreciate everything that pink has to offer. I love its soft, relaxing, calm tone on one end of the scale and its bright, enthusiastic boldness on the other. My house has been thoughtfully decorated with a little bit of pink in many rooms for years. Shortly after my diagnosis, my daughter was home visiting from college. Standing in our home while struggling to sort through her feelings, she said pink was all she could see around her. Pink had now changed in meaning. Some days, even a little pink ribbon can be too much for those still struggling through this journey. What was created to be supportive is sometimes a sad reminder of an unwelcome new identity and of the fact that normalcy would never return to our lives as we once knew it.

I was on a prescheduled hospital stay out of state. To fill my day between appointments, I would add the suggested activities offered throughout the day to relieve stress from all the health appointments. I participated in the art session, which was intended to provide some therapy. Around the long tables sat patients and caregivers side by side, all engaged in the task at hand. The assignment was to paint what cancer felt like. *OK*, I thought, *give me a brush. But I do not think there are enough ugly colors I can spread around this canvas to help you understand what that word feels like to me.*

It must have helped my mind somehow because I never forgot my picture. It was not one that would win an award or appear on a quilt square, but it was helpful to my process—a pink road, which signified a journey, that took a turn into a gray mass that went black and then faded back to a permanent cloudy deep gray. That was what I thought cancer felt like: an awful disruption, a confusing commotion, a dismal disorder. My picture began to erode in places where I kept dragging the brush, and somehow, I could not get the colors dark enough on the canvas.

Months later, I saw the winning paintings published in a coffee table book at that same hospital. The elaborate creations were thoughtful, beautiful, and in step with all the feelings I related to but could not communicate. I could not understand how someone who had cancer could create something so meaningful out of the darkness, but they had. Several of them had and the results were complex and beautifully stunning.

There were award-winning, intricate designs carefully created to illustrate the same feelings through which I was journeying. Those artists were able to hone their skills and use this challenge and their emotions to bring resolve. That, I could appreciate and relate to.

YOUNG

My doctors initially told me I was younger than the determined acceptable age to get breast cancer. No other explanation. Statistics indicated I was too young. I had no more understanding or insight but learned that identifying the "too young" category meant more aggressive care, a preselected course of treatment, and a longer lifespan to focus on preserving.

Given no space to refute my willingness or question the effectiveness of these strongly suggested recommendations, I bought it. I bought the big-ticket chemotherapy, the life-altering six and a half weeks of radioactive pulses that would forever change me, and now the commitment of a lifetime of hormone-altering medications that would reshape my health. As a result, I now had the after-purchase regret and frustration of making such huge decisions under duress without the time needed to learn and consider all the facts.

Both my oncologists were young—younger than me—new, and in hindsight, likely underexperienced. Amid the whirlwind of information, I never considered the sources: who they were, what they knew or did not know, and why they made the referrals or had the responses they did. I believed that everyone must know more than me on the subject, and I did not consider enough or challenge the information. All I could manage to do was sit attentively in the moment and try to take in as much of the data as I could.

Who can rationally weigh out and thoughtfully consider each portion and source? I was already under so much pressure to understand this information and make the best decision possible. On the outside, I looked accepting and agreeable, but on the inside, I felt crumpled with a steady flow of unnerving fear.

I never asked about experience or past practices or reviewed the credentials on the wall. I listened, I took most of it in, and I made what few decisions were lightly presented from the three scenarios that were relayed to me, which all included some combination of chemotherapy, medication, and radiation.

Five months after the radiation ended, and frustrated at the conclusion of the treatments, I began to look for more than had been offered to me originally. I wanted reliable information, dependable insight, and a thorough understanding of the disease and its effects. I sought care options that would promote restoration and bring health to what was now damage to many parts of my body. I wanted to feel strong again and figure out how what had been broken could be repaired and restored.

Not everything is a conspiracy, but because some things are, I wanted assurance that I was not just a statistic or part of an experiment. I had watched the occasional (OK, more than occasional during my surgery recoveries) documentary and then at once cut out mistreated beef from my diet and refused to buy another bottle of misrepresented water. With the uncertain outcome I had been left with, I wanted to be practical and informed as I unpacked real and significant concerns.

I had filed away in my brain the stories of the two Lisas and other strong survivors I had met along the way, patients whom I witnessed actively participating in both their own care and prognosis. I read victorious testimonials from formerly incurable patients, met people with turnaround stories, and learned of years of life and hope that had been restored.

In discovering the practices and methods of other countries and in viewing videos and lectures, weighing statistics, considering lifestyle changes, and listening to traditional medicine advocates, I was able to find the type of help I could easily understand, make sense of, and live with. Multiple resources gave me new understanding that harsh drugs were not the only answer.

We find ourselves only a click away from an onslaught of verifiable information from sources around the globe. Some of the information I found was good, some of it questionable, and some of it dangerously unsupported. Judging the look and feel of a source did not always authenticate a hopeful and better conclusion, but repetition—finding the same information from multiple sources—did.

I learned as much as I could, sometimes asking the same questions others had. Research gave me some power over my situation, helped me guard my individuality, and reminded me that there were options and choices I did have.

I wanted to understand my care, my situation, and my alternatives outside the limited responses I had received or what I had been told was "common protocol." I cautiously challenged the theories I read about, not pretending to know anything more than I knew or be anything more than who I was. But what if there were more approaches than what I had been told of? I was not a doctor, but this was my body, which was too important to treat casually or to trust to everyone.

There was evidence that healthy diets, vitamins, and supplements were effective. Exercise would make a difference, despite the exhaustion I felt throughout my body. There were documented statistics from reputable foundations that said healing could happen. There were new alternatives and ways to get out from underneath the lifetime of medicine and the "medicine is all that is necessary" dialogue I had been listening to.

There was also too much evidence that the medical community I had been leaning on for all my answers may have failed to deliver the complete and best scenario—whole care. If you have cancer, take your medicine, but know that there is a lot more you can do to help yourself. Natural supplements, nutritional support, healthy lifestyle changes, and vitamins build your strength and stamina. You can regain energy, have peace of mind, and sleep soundly again. Being a part of a faith community also builds hope and can provide a healthy support network.

This journey of exploration and discovery empowered me, giving me a sense of control over my body and my health, and renewed my hope for the future. Pausing and focusing on self-care options can go a long way toward sorting out the lies from the truth and making a strong comeback. This self-care journey brought me relief and peace of mind, helping me better understand and address my individual needs. As I found my way through the heaviness, my ability to problem-solve and advocate for myself began to improve.

I saw a mental picture of myself just as I was in a photo from when I was a young child. I was wearing an ironed blue dress and had an innocent smile on my face. I was bravely standing on top of a huge mountain and suddenly associated that mountain with cancer. How had that girl found her way up there? How could she have ever known what was coming or ever been prepared? Conquering such a daunting mountain could only happen with strength, determination, and hope. This climb was an all-consuming journey to unfamiliar high places, and I needed a map I did not have.

While mountain climbing, it can be intimidating and overwhelming to look at what is ahead. When you do get to the top, you realize you are OK, and you might think, *I might have been able to keep climbing longer if I needed to.* On that high mountaintop, things change. The climb, now completed, looks different from when you started. You have gained a new perspective, understanding, and appreciation. You have arrived, and you are still you.

Something changes when you finish something you could not imagine completing. The same mountain you had to climb is the one that would be unfathomable to those around you because they have told you as much. You realize that the young girl is still inside and that since you still have that innocent smile, this experience has not taken what it threatened and has not ruined you as promised. You have arrived on top. The climb is over, and desperation and unbelief are now behind you.

At least for this part of the journey, you have done what others did not believe they could ever do. You can smile again, and there is still an innocence there. You are better off for having walked with a struggle than having sat down and quit. You have a new balance, a new perspective, renewed endurance, and stronger feet that carry you farther than you ever knew. Things that used to derail you seem so much smaller in the wake of a life-threatening journey. This transforming season left a bold new perspective and a strong sense of hope for my future.

I can promise that in the face of cancer, inside you grows a new yearning to do those things that you have placed on hold, saved for a later date, not believed possible, or let stop you along the way. You will get to the top of your mountain with a sense of abandon inside you to live your life fully. Regret becomes an ugly word that suddenly means you may have run out of opportunities to finish or try.

I am not sure when it all morphed into something new for me. Little by little, I considered that where I was walking was dangerous and that I could lose my life. Maybe it was all at once, or perhaps it came slowly as I marked treatment-ending anniversaries on the calendar. All I can be sure of now and confidently convey is that I am not the same person I was before. This process changed me, and in hindsight, I can confidently claim it was for the better.

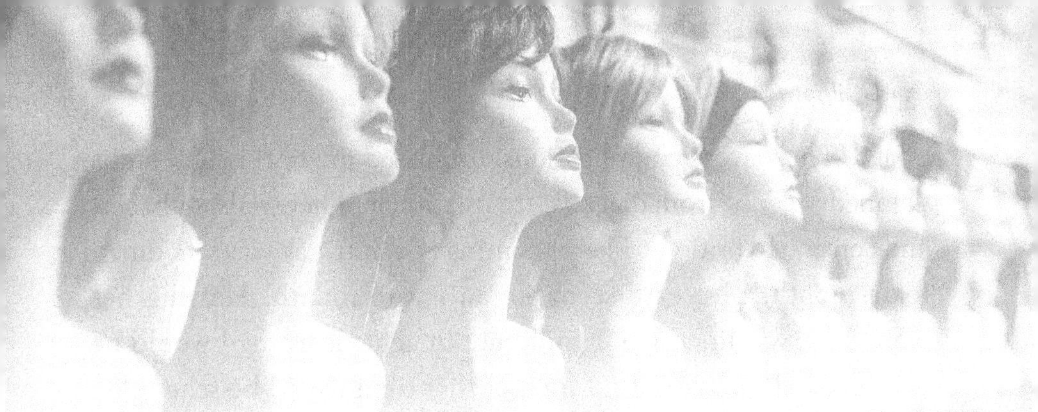

FRIENDS

Through my research, I have discovered a medical group at a cancer hospital that agreed to take over all my care. I travel out of state on a schedule for screenings, treatments, and support, and a team collaborates behind the scenes to keep me healthy. Each scheduled trip involves exploring opportunities, options, and new choices in my care. They have helped me to understand my health, and I have confidence in their ability to address my individualized needs.

Once I found them and experienced this difference, I could let my guard down and stop searching. I am on a new journey, witnessing amazing stories from other patients because I have found a dedicated team, a community, and a strategy I can trust. They are committed to missing nothing, and I have never looked back or regretted the change I made in treatment.

I made two new friends while loading the airport van for my drive to the airport from the cancer treatment hospital. The first was an elementary school teacher with career-ending ovarian cancer who had been newly diagnosed. Her doctor insisted she no longer be around children regularly because of germs. Ushered quickly into an unexpected early retirement, she began chemotherapy, and life as she had previously known it suddenly ended. There were complications, unrelated medical issues, and a detailed account from diagnosis to treatment of her trials, setbacks, and continued options. Her upcoming hospital stay was scheduled for a month. Best-case scenario, an entire month! Hearing her words overwhelmed me. I could not imagine learning I would be in a hospital for a month. Much of that time would be scheduled in intensive care, addressing the most serious concerns, with a follow-up on the regular care floor monitoring any complications.

She and I shared in-depth for the next few hours during the van ride and the walk through the airport, then finally we hugged goodbye outside the women's room for our parting flights. I never found out her name, and I find it ironic that we shared so many details of our intimate medical histories and personal stories without ever introducing ourselves. Hers was an account of cancer I could not easily forget. I wished her well and committed to praying for her, and I did, but not by name. God knows her name and had our paths cross for a reason.

As I think about her situation, I cannot imagine the whirlwind of changes she faced and the things she was immediately forced to give up. Her career, years of work with children, and likely her passion was gone because of a situation she could not have prepared for or seen coming. I wondered about her support system and how her life may have suddenly shifted. I prayed that she would be anchored to lifelines critical to her success and that the grace would be given to her to manage those new transitions.

My next friend was small, and although she was very personable and friendly, she was quite feisty and, from what I could tell, unbreakable in spirit. She had to be. She had undetected blood cancer that had already spread to many of her major organs. It was found only after her multiple and mostly ignored demands for a thorough scan two years prior. "Not enough indicators"; "It is probably nothing"; "There is no family history"; "Your insurance denied the authorization." The doctor filtered the excuses to her one by one, and as she recounted those challenging conversations, I found it unthinkable to imagine the frustration of not being heard. She knew her body, knew something was wrong, and with unshakable determination, kept asking for help but was not listened to—an unbelievable story to hear, but not so much anymore.

We are becoming conditioned to accept that health insurance is not an automatic safety net of people cheering for your best care when you are facing your worst moments. They are not there to catch your concerns and ensure your future. You are a statistic, a risk calculated by how many in your bloodline have proven to be afflicted and survived the same cellular anomaly.

This woman said she had begged and bargained with her doctor. "If you do the scan, I will honor any life changes you request." The regretful doctor apologized profusely as he walked back in and said he had been utterly wrong. There were spots everywhere on the scan. "You only have weeks left to live," he solemnly said.

"No," she said, "I am going to fight this."

"You are amazing," he replied after a somber pause. And she was. She had to get up every day and fight. She had an adopted eight-year-old at home, and she felt she had no choice but to fight. All the odds were against her; there was no cure, no predetermined way, no better diagnosis around the corner, and no hopeful promises. It was up to her to decide why she had come, and it was up to her not to go home until she knew she was finished.

Fight cancer. I never understood what that phrase even meant. I saw it branded across bumpers and chests alike. I even understood that the pink swish stood for the fight. How does one, or a thousand, fight? In the corner of my mind, I was beginning to collect an understanding of what it looked like to fight cancer through the unique and challenged individuals who were relentlessly doing it every day.

Sometimes, it meant getting up and continuing to participate in the therapy, the medicines, the appointments, and the subsequent surgery. For others, the focus was on a positive attitude against a predetermined outcome. And for some, it was saying yes to the treatment one more day despite how it made them feel. It also meant a targeted focus on some much-needed self-care and sometimes justifying choosing the cheesecake because, after all, you have cancer. And besides, chemo has made you suddenly lose weight (again, not by your own design).

But for me, fighting cancer meant that I began to frequent health food stores and learn about the power of vitamins and herbal compounds. It meant that a once simple decision to grab something to eat now had become a search for something with the nutritional value and the amount of protein my body required. It meant listening to five other people in the row on the airplane ordering the same junk food and my wanting to explain to them the importance of guarding their health. It meant hours of searching online to understand terms and treatments and learn about new options.

It was also the distraction of a sudden spasm or shooting pain and the wonder of what could be next. It was the handful of medications and supplements in the morning that dictated that skipping breakfast was not an option. Those same pills caused a great deal of nausea in an empty stomach. It meant the frantic purchase of a juicer with the hope that I would gain a new desire for vegetable juice. It was the pregnant stall in front of the mirror: hat, scarf, or wig—*or am I ready to step out bald?*—and the self-destructive thoughts that followed. It was new routines, new obstacles, and a brand-new normal. It was following the schedule of supplements, medications, and appointments and finding the necessary focus it took to manage it all.

Fighting cancer meant taking a walk when I wanted to do nothing and resting when I needed to do other things. It was the lopsided feeling in a plain old T-shirt and the new reality that only one type of bra would ever really work again with my now complicated shape. It meant swapping my thoughts, the bad for the good. And as a pastor reminded me, it was about making room for the truth instead of solely believing the facts told to me. It was learning to ask for and then accept help. It also meant accepting that things would not get done the way I would have done them and that I could not do anything about it. No amount of worry would change that. It meant deliberately denying some stress, or at least trying to. It meant keeping an eye on my hidden guilt meter that jumped with the unrealistic blame for bringing a painful journey of cancer to my family. And when I came to the end of myself, it was learning to let go and let God in because only He could quiet the hearts of my loved ones and soothe their fears. After all, I was in line for the same help they needed from Him.

ACT

"What can I do to help?"

I have few answers right now. I do not know what you can do, because I am still trying to figure out what I can, should, or should not do. All the things that you want to do to help would be welcome. I would not reject and would applaud any help you want to give.

Sure, when a friend brought an enchilada casserole to our door, it may not have seemed as significant to him, but it surprised me and put a lump in my throat. It was only days after we had learned about and were trying to cope with my diagnosis. The knock on the door and the visit was unexpected but welcomed. Beyond the meal, I knew he loved my family and wanted to do something. I imagined him thinking of us and our situation and setting aside the other things in his day to cook this meal. It meant so much more than the small thank-you that I said that day. We reveled in the food, the company, and the heart of friendship behind the act.

So, my advice to everyone and anyone who knows someone who has been diagnosed with cancer is to do something. Make a meal, make a phone call, send a card, say a prayer. No act of love will go unnoticed or be unnecessary in the uncertain shadow of cancer.

I had two kids in college at the time of my diagnosis, and one of them was out of state. The one out of state had always managed the six-hundred-mile distance from home without any problems. She was strong and independent, and she navigated all aspects of her college life well. When 0.8 millimeters in diameter was added to that number, things that previously had never been a challenge suddenly became hard.

Nothing I could say could reassure my daughter, because this was happening to me. She held back her questions, feelings, sadness, and fears to keep from being more demanding on me. She processed her thoughts alone, quietly, and isolated from her family. I could do nothing about it. Cancer was also a new walk for me, and I had no idea what could help or hinder her need to process.

Years later, I learned that late one night at college, she was no longer able to stuff it all inside. After having run out of space to push down those feelings, she let down her guard and confided in a friend. Thankfully, she had someone close by who was willing to listen at the most crucial time for her when she finally needed to share it.

Nobody at any age is ready to manage an unexpected presence of cancer. One way to help is to reach out to the kids who are struggling to process and grab their new reality. They have no skills or experience, no promise it will end well, and no help. They often get overlooked, standing on the sidelines with a mountain of feelings and facts they do not understand and are powerless to navigate. Their silence, game face, or anger should be understood as the fear that this situation knowingly produces. I do not think I would have ever known how critical it is to attend to the children unless I had gone through it myself and watched the effects firsthand.

If ever there is another person close to me going through a similar challenge, I will remember to include reaching out to the kids in my plans. They need critical lifelines in the form of reassurance, understanding and stability. Do something, anything, because now they need everything.

Two years later, one of my kids had a friend whose mother died of cancer, and the reality once again came crashing down. From a deep unhealed wound, she unpacked the feelings and raw memories from the day she first heard my diagnosis. The memory of where she was and what she was doing when I had to tell her was being relived, that moment when I pulled her unexpectedly into a place no teenager should have had to go. Unfairly, and unexpectedly again, she was processing a layer of hurt, and all I could do was comfort her and reassure her that it was not her story. I have raised independent, confident kids, but nobody can be prepared for a mass that challenges the comfort and peace of a predictable life.

One weekend after treatments had started, my sisters arranged to bring a takeout meal over to our house for dinner. We sat on the floor in our living room, ate, talked, and played games. Nobody mentioned cancer or asked any questions. They did not need to. Cancer was why we were there. They had taken the time to plan this and be there with me and their support spoke volumes.

It could be that no one else remembers that day, but I do. I remember how they organized it and what restaurant they brought the food from, all because it was attached to an act of love. It is a simple but comforting memory I will always fondly remember.

The day after Mother's Day, I was driving to work and noticed caramel on my sweater sleeve from making popcorn for my family the night before. A spot that years ago would have caused me to focus on changing clothes, was now satisfying. At that moment, I was reminded that I would not trade the stains, the challenges, or the exhaustion from cooking, cleaning, or caring. I am committed to my family and mindful of giving, preparing, and offering my best. Like everybody, I have days of wanting a break, but that feeling quickly disappears when I realize I am the one made to soothe, help, and rescue. Today, I have the opportunity to have the role of a mom. I love my role and take it on gratefully because nobody, including me, is promised tomorrow.

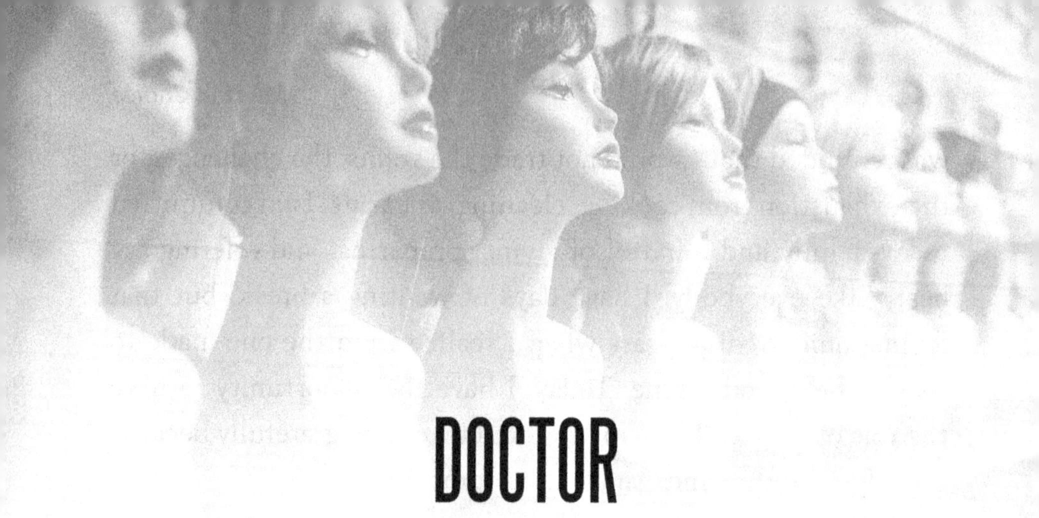

DOCTOR

The yearly exam, intended to be routine, was scheduled to ensure the medicine was not causing any hidden adverse side effects. I never guessed a small discussion after an annual exam would have ended here. It brought another biopsy that would cause a phone call two days later. And once again, it was the worst-case scenario. I had become one of the 2 or 3 percent (I can no longer remember the statistics. The number is written down somewhere in the file I keep with the biology reports from early on).

There were cell changes, and they were not good. Cancer statistics were cited, and the impending prognosis was relayed to me in matter-of-fact terms that were difficult to hear. The time for these cells to present as a new cancer was varied and unpredictable but very sure to happen as I had just been warned. This would not go away or resolve on its own, and now I heard that once again, the only choice being explained to me was to accept the plan.

"We need to remove everything, and I am recommending a radical hysterectomy. Uterus, ovaries, and fallopian tubes are for cycles, which you are done with, and for carrying babies, which you no longer need to do." I heard the shocking stream of words come from the doctor's mouth, and they oddly echoed in my head as I sat motionless and unable to speak. *Wait. Stop. This is going too fast again, and you are not me,* I think. She barely paused to breathe as she continued to callously deliver the factual version of her unapologetic findings. I was visibly trying to manage the shock wave of terms just used to dismantle my body. What the doctor was saying was medically accurate, but so bottom line for her to say.

As she spoke, I felt my stomach tighten as flashbacks of chemo began to race through my mind. I admired her self-confidence and assertiveness. I knew she was not there to talk about how this made me feel, but was she even considering how this was making me feel? Each of those organs, my organs, had a purpose, had a connection, and was part of me. She was verbally disposing of them rapidly and hastily without considering the immense impact of her words.

The doctor was referring to the half pound of tissue that dictated the pink "It's a girl" name card on my hospital bassinet. The same organs that identified me meant I might cry easily also meant I might not be able to stand up to my brothers and caused me to have a sensitive side. I had waited anxiously at twelve years old to see if those same organs would predictably produce eggs, and now they would be gone in the two hours she said it would take to remove them.

In one long thought, the doctor described her coworker, her upcoming schedule opening, and her confidence in her colleague's surgery skills. Meanwhile, I was sitting there with the same astonished expression on my face, trying to manage the findings. Her pace, approach, and recklessness demolished any faith I had gained in her qualifications and care. I was two long years into this cancer journey and a bit wiser now. I wanted a second source to give me the same recommendation before I would be ready to head down the path this doctor said was inevitable.

Holding my thick file in her hands, the doctor was aware of

my history. Just because that folder was comprehensive did not mean that she should have assumed I was prepared for another distressing diagnosis. I knew she had been practicing her game face for years, but she must have seen the look on my face and the dismay in my eyes. This news removed the peace in my life that I had only recently gathered again. I worked hard to listen and ask intelligent questions, but this time, I was slowing this entire process down to a more comfortable speed.

Significant life changes were happening, and I had a focus on family that needed to remain guarded in this season. Coming up was a well-deserved college graduation that we were getting ready to celebrate. I could not imagine unfairly stealing the attention because of my health once again. Adding another surprise surgery and recuperation period to a busy family life and a full-time career seemed impossible, let alone the new medication changes with serious new side effects that she also stated would be inevitable. It was an awful surprise start-over that I deemed very unwelcome.

Most importantly, I did not want to introduce any more uncertainty, fear, stress, or worry to anyone around me. I wished not to have come for that appointment, heard of her findings, or realized anything was going wrong in my body again. I wanted a better picture and more information to feel that I had choices and different options. I felt powerless to stop this all-consuming train coming straight at me. Despite the doctor's offer to send in the scheduler, I did not have time during the opening in her calendar in two weeks to completely change my life again.

It had only been a few years of my faithfully taking the long-term medication I had already been told was my only option. It had already been an ongoing challenge to stay on the medicine while navigating the consequences from chemotherapy and radiation. I had been juggling and sorting out unforeseen side effects from multiple sources. Prescriptions typically have side effects, but I believed the list should be smaller, and the percentages and number of people afflicted minimal. I never considered how many would appear or that when they did, it would bring me to this place again of being backed into a corner.

I had been reminded at every appointment to stay on this treatment course despite the side effects. The list of risks was long and included ovarian cancer, which was an obvious head-scratcher for me. The only alternative seemed disobedient or dismissive: to walk away from all follow-up care despite every well-educated professional recommendation. Each option seemed just as negligent as the other, and each was not good in the face of reoccurring cancer. I had no business creating my own care plan, but I felt there had to be a better way. I vowed to find another option and set out to look for more answers.

I boarded a plane for a second opinion from a different surgeon at a cancer treatment hospital. He agreed with the same suggested course of surgery to remove the organs and begin the new medication. The facts remained that the cell changes were present, predictable and unfavorable. I was not surprised by his recommendations, as I know surgeons are trained to end risk by cutting.

With the second opinion, I was ready to trust this doctor that assured me that this was the best response for the least chance of cancer recurrence. I had come to the end of my efforts to seek better options and succumbed to the only plan I now knew. My organs were removed surgically by a robotic arm, and like clockwork, I began a new recovery period as a new hormone-altering medication was added to my daily routine. Once again, I began to navigate the new harsh side effects as I pushed away feelings of loss and disappointment. My health continued to feel out of control and at risk.

HEROES

She walked boldly up to the oncology desk and gave her name to the nurse as she very confidently checked herself in. "Never stop fighting" was written on the back of a red satin cape that she proudly wore over her street clothes. Sad, the cape looked worn and a little old. She had noticeably been fighting for a while—too long, I imagined. I noticed her because of her age and remarkable confidence, and with that, she seemed unusually comfortable in this scene. With thin brown hair and a small frame with a slight build, she could not have been more than sixteen years old.

A tired mom trailed a few steps behind, carrying all their belongings. The mother's face was weary and cast a worried look, with lines that appeared where a smile most likely used to be. Purses, bags, a pillow, and too much paperwork filled the mother's arms. They had each practiced these roles many times and no longer needed to communicate their actions to one another as they arrived at appointment after appointment.

My eyes scanned the room. Sitting by himself was "face in hands," rubbing his eyes repeatedly as if to erase what he had seen or dreaded seeing. Next to him was "awkward wheelchair," rolling back and forth, struggling to find a place to park, along with a caregiver fumbling to assist. There were common characteristics everywhere I looked: sunken faces, listless eyes, shaky hands, and unstable feet. Across the room, a child sat next to a parent, each appearing miles away, lost on the devices they held in their hands. This would be the most unreasonable place and the most unreasonable situation to insist on others being present in conversation even after traveling here to join you. Headphones, movies, emails, and texting were all practical escapes from the current heaviness looming in the room.

Young with old, husband with wife, child with parent, parent with child. This room did not discriminate between any group or subset. Ginger ale, crackers, warm blankets, sickness bags, and knitted hats were graciously offered around every corner. You were either here to push the wheelchair or to be the one riding in it. There were no sentimental scenes here of couples walking side by side, healthy and carefree. Generously offered stress balls, magazines, partially completed puzzles, and pages to color, and loosely facilitated games, giveaways, and gatherings, were around every corner. Distractions, distractions, distractions.

This was the big league, a daunting picture you never wanted to find yourself part of. This was the bump in the road, the big bump everyone feared; the detour no one ever expected; the rugged mountain named cancer these people unexpectedly found themselves climbing, straight uphill with no map or warning.

Those with any focus or energy left were distracted by the TVs in the room or the clipboards of paperwork in their hands, slumping in chairs until they heard their names called. From waiting area to waiting area, wheelchairs, pillows, and IV poles were being toted around. Eyes were uncontrollably moving up and down, noticing patient wristbands, caregiver name tags, weakness, worry, hair loss, and fragility. To a patient, it could feel like being in a fishbowl with all eyes on the obvious. There was nowhere to hide, and strangers one could not help but notice were inspecting each other intently.

For everyone, there was no privacy and no question about the reason we were here. Cancer had intruded into the lives of everyone present in this place. Visitors to this hospital and those unfamiliar with this treatment environment were overly courteous and anxiously willing to help in any small way. They wanted to show their empathy and support, but most were at a loss as to how.

Masks always made sense here, but then any smiles got missed, were overlooked, or were poignantly, consciously restricted. There was no trusted map, no one-size-fits-all best practice, and no natural course or method. Every person pooled in this scene was figuring it out step by step, moment by moment, need by need. Cancer did not fit well anywhere for anyone. Nobody taking steps through this diagnosis was assured they were on the correct path. These were trials, and trials commonly come with plenty of pressure and no guarantees.

No wonder that young girl had chosen such a bright superhero cape to mask her thin failing body. It is only her in this fight. It is up to her, and she is the fight. You go, girl, all the way to the finish line in that satin cape and anything else you decide is necessary for this season. If clothes, a wild hat, or zany socks make you feel strong, then wear 'em proud. Those are your coping tools, your personality identifiers, and yes, your armor in this extraordinarily long, confusing, and turbulent season.

Undoubtedly, she had to leave much behind to grow up overnight and manage all aspects of this incredibly damaging and untimely life interruption. There was a complete focus on everything medical and on cells that cannot be seen that were uprooting her youth and normalcy.

These should have been her carefree years with friends,

shopping, and trivial worries, but they were not. She had been medically tackled and derailed at such an early age. The list of what she had given up, having had to learn all too well the terms, treatments, side effects, and unfortunately, her own prognosis, was exceptionally long and unfair. Forced to be all in, she had no guarantee of an end in sight, and I was sad to see her young face, an all too familiar occurrence in this place.

I heard my name suddenly called, and I snapped back to the reality that I, too, was here for similar reasons. I followed the technician down the hall and thought, *Here I am again—the same routine.* I had lost count of what number mammogram this was. I found myself in this familiar room filled with the same sickening uncertainty. With my clothing off and my drafty gown open in the front, I stood facing the machine as I began pondering what would happen next.

The lights were dimmed, and there was some faint background music, but nothing about this was relaxing or comforting. The heavy, clear acrylic plates come down, and the machine begins to whir loudly as it painfully compresses every bit of breast tissue into a flattened, thin mass void of form, hoping to illuminate anything ominous.

Nothing about this process felt feminine, dignified, or humane. There was nowhere else to look beside the scarred tissue painfully pulled from my chest that appeared oddly spilled between the plates. "Picture looks good," the technician said, but I had heard that before. Her words indicated the test was over and I felt relief. It would be some time before I learned the truth and had the results explained in a few words or with fractions of particles described in hundredths. *This scenario is now what it will always look like,* I thought. There was no escaping this scene, which will inevitably play over and over again for years to come.

Getting dressed again, I noticed the only sign in the room: "Be the change you wish to see in the world." OK, I thought, *give me time, energy, and my focus back. I will be the change, cause the change, or do all the changes; I just need the time.*

AFTERMATH

I had the same nightmare again last night. The cancer had come back with a fury. The images and the overwhelming rush of emotions felt real. I panicked as I watched myself walking through it. The pain, despair, and anguish once again disrupted everything. It was not the cancer itself that was the hardest, but all that it did to the people I loved. I began the conversations all over again. I watched it like a movie as my news again devastated those lives.

Cancer is a destroyer. It stops life and shadows everything else in its reach. It knocks on any door, respects nobody, and knocks everything else to the ground for the moment. But then there is God. I woke up and told my husband about the nightmare, and he told me, "God already healed you," in a sympathetic but conclusive tone. The images, my heart racing, and the sick and sinking feelings began to subside.

The truth is that God did heal me. I could not imagine getting through that season without Him rescuing me from every dark thought and bringing me through every challenge. God changed me and how I thought about cancer. It was no longer a mountain in front of me but one I looked over fearlessly with triumphant confidence.

God did not heal me as I had hoped for. Through most of this journey, I felt weak, faithless, and distracted without hope and with little optimism. No miraculous test results caused a team of doctors to gather around and be astonished that a tumor had suddenly disappeared. It did not happen all at once.

Instead, God used surgeons, supplements, support, and time. There was no shortcut or rushing through the process. Any movement felt like baby steps. He was patient with me; it took practice and endurance to build my faith and feel restored on the other side of the circumstances.

I am not better or worse than someone else who has cancer as part of their story. I realize how lonely, dark, and desolate the unknown path of cancer can feel. There are no guaranteed methods, paths, or promises. It is about day-to-day questions, trials, decisions, and results. I relinquished thinking I had power over all those situations. But that did not make me immune to the struggles, the illness, or the threats that the illness can bring.

When I came home from the first long day of chemotherapy, I was understandably worn out. Cautioned that in a matter of hours my body would begin to decline rapidly from the harsh treatment, I watched and waited. I was on a strict schedule of medications around the clock. I set up everything I would need in front of the TV and was grateful the day was over. I did my best to rest and put it all behind me.

Faith had always been a foundational part of our family, but I had no idea what I needed, so my hopeless prayers were short desperate random cries for help. My son unexpectedly told me that he wanted to pray for my chemo to end, an idea I had no space even to consider or grasp on my own. I did not know if it was his or God's idea, so I dismissed it only as his compassion, but I agreed. He prayed for me, and I returned to waiting and watching.

The next day, I began to develop signs of an allergic reaction to the drugs, and my oncologist canceled all remaining future infusions. That was the end of chemotherapy for me, and I never had to go back. I recently learned that one of the same drugs I took is now causing serious, permanent damage to some patients. Patients are now casualties of the same treatments that promised to bring help and do good.

I never accepted cancer for the damage and destruction that it causes. Instead, I assumed that it meant treatments I had not planned on, interruptions I did not see coming, and medications I did not like. Some freedom came from changing my perspective and accepting what I could not change. It has been a long journey, but I am not afraid of cancer any longer. I have learned to find a positive purpose on the other side of all that pain.

TESTIMONY

I hosted a luncheon for the young women from our church. They were college students and had been positive role models for our young girls and many others. We always valued any opportunity to spend time with them and honor them. I planned a special tea party to show them how appreciated they were. I had prepared to host this event a year before, but we had difficulty aligning our schedules with this busy group.

I knew as I was preparing for this day that God was putting it on my heart to share my cancer journey. Until now, I had only shared one-on-one and never gave all the details. Despite these faces being familiar, I felt vulnerable sharing such an intimate story in front of any group. I conceded to the idea and wrote out my story, knowing I would need to rely heavily on my scripted words to stay on track from start to finish.

I prepared our dining room with an extra-long table covered in linens and mismatched floral china teacups with silver table settings. The scene was beautiful and elegant just as I had pictured. As we poured tea and passed around platters of mini sandwiches, cookies, and cakes, there was lots of laughter and heartfelt sharing. But as we talked, I secretly felt sick and nervous as my speaking time quickly approached. I pulled a high stool up to the end of the long table to see each of the nineteen faces to the end. I sat down with my notes and my only prop, a flowered box with a tassel closure.

I swallowed the lump in my throat as I prepared to share my story. I got everyone's attention and slowly and methodically began reading about my journey. "As I was planning this day," I started, "God began to speak to me about this box. Sharing it is difficult because I have not had to tell my story or be honest about how this cancer battle has felt. Speaking in front of a group and being open about my feelings are two things I am the least comfortable doing, and today, I feel called to do both."

I continued speaking without pause. "About two years ago, I was diagnosed with breast cancer. I was not sick, and there was no history of breast cancer in my family. I was unprepared for any diagnosis like this. But let me tell you how good God was right from the start. I knew something was up as God repeatedly prompted me to get an overdue mammogram. I knew when I scheduled that first appointment and then got the call back to have it redone that something was already wrong. I knew when I got the biopsy done and before the doctor was honest with me that she suspected it was cancer. And I knew as I was led into the oversized dressing room, followed by a very motherly nurse, that God was with me."

I began to explain the mammograms, the biopsy, the conversations, and the phone calls. My story was flowing as I recounted surgeries, healing periods, revelations, struggles, and promises. I continued explaining my experiences on chemo day and how much my husband's support had helped. I talked about what the chemo did to my body and how desperate I felt having to have my ponytail cut off. I explained how strange it was not to have eyebrows, eyelashes, or hair on my legs for months after the treatment.

I looked up briefly, and to my surprise, every face was solemn, sympathetic, and extremely focused. My words seemed to matter to them, and I was grateful in that moment that I was willing to let God use my testimony to touch their hearts. I was beginning to understand the importance of sharing it as I listened to myself recount the long journey.

It was finally time to reveal the contents of the box that had been sitting on my lap. I carefully opened the box and lifted my ponytail with the hair tie still intact. "In this box is the ponytail that was cut off while I sat on the bathroom floor that day. Looking at it, I remember being at the beginning of a battle that I had no idea how it would end. I watched cancer hurt those around me and cause all of us to struggle. I learned to keep looking at God and coming to Him, especially when I was scared and did not know what to do or say.

Some things have changed for me after having gone through this. I trust God more and worry less. Cancer does not loom over my life anymore. I relinquish control of my plans a lot easier than I used to. I am more patient and more appreciative of my family. I stop, look at my life, and remember to feel grateful."

As I neared the end, I shared with them, "God has continued to remind me of this box and some small keys I had purchased a year ago to decorate for this same event. He told me to write down and attach to each key a promise I learned through this experience and to give one to each of you. These keys, each with an individualized personal message, have been placed under your plates. I prayed that each of you would sit where the promise was that you needed to here today."

The room was quiet as they lifted their plates and found their key. Each young woman read her message privately. By their expressions and the thoughtful contemplation on each face, I could tell that they had received the promise they needed that day. There were tears in the eyes of daughters, neighbors, and friends, all of whom had been affected by a cancer diagnosis and story.

I listened to their stories and what the messages that accompanied their respective keys meant to each of them. Their experiences were weighty and varied, but somehow this story connected with each of them. One young woman had a mom who had breast cancer when she was young, and she was learning insight she had never known. One young woman said she now knew what type of nurse she wanted to be: an oncology nurse.

There are no words for knowing God had used me to impart powerful lessons that made such an impact. I follow the one who wanted to be an oncology nurse on social media, and she accomplished just that. She did what she felt called to do, and I am sure it will impact the world.

PROMISES

These are the lessons from God that I learned in the face of cancer and that I attached to those keys. I have no more words except to share these powerful and everlasting promises. Please covet each one of them as your own.

- God is always with me.
- God is always in control.
- Trust the Holy Spirit.
- I am His; He cares for me.
- He has good plans for me.
- He is everything I need.
- He will never leave me.
- He gives me hope.
- I can trust Him.
- He will lead me.
- He will lift me up.
- He will give me what I need.
- My strength comes from Him.
- He is my strong tower.
- He has healing for me.
- I hear His voice.
- He is close to me.
- He is jealous for me.
- God knows.

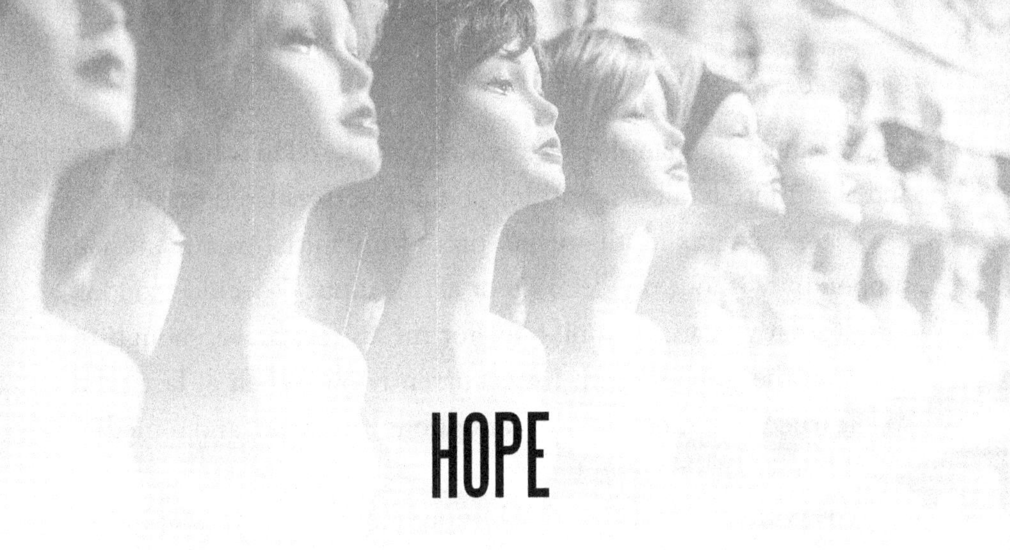

HOPE

My first oncologist told my husband that taking vitamins would not positively affect my health. Although she did not put it as eloquently as that, her answer was dismissive and misinformed. Being educated and health-conscious, my husband disagreed with her methodology. Having lost faith in my care, he began quietly looking for more resources and options. Stuffing his genuine opinions, he waited until I was ready for a change in care.

After several months of following along with my head down and doing everything the doctors said, I began to question if there was more. When the same professional could not steer me toward any helpful resources or offer me any hope, it was time for me to seek different answers.

I had a false sense of trust in my first oncologist. Because she was female, I had expected her to advocate more, pursue my best interests, and tirelessly root for my care. Surely, she must have known that I was an individual. She had breasts, hair, and feelings and would be aware of the loss I was experiencing.

As I looked back at my circumstances, I found no evidence that my doctor had considered the person behind the cells, the chemicals, and the diagnosis. I realized she was merely signing off on the same care plan she routinely administered to other patients and that there had been nothing about it personalized for me.

After recognizing that every part of my initial treatment had slipped by without my decision or active input, I decided to look for alternative care. It took a lot for me to feel brave enough to question the medical path I was currently on. When at last I did so, I learned that there were other options, therapies, and remedies that I knew nothing about.

It was then that I found a comprehensive cancer hospital in another state that was willing to take over my care with a sense of confident urgency that I had not yet experienced during this illness. The facility is widely accessible and, very importantly, does not appear to discriminate against income or diagnosis. Through this comprehensive care, I have been offered help from nutritionists, counselors, naturopaths, and various therapists—a complete team I never could have assembled on my own.

My cancer treatment now includes research specialists who meet to study my case, evaluate my health from every angle, review my scans, discuss my clinical diagnosis, and make the necessary next-step plans. My treatments, recommendations, and doctor notes are all pooled in one accessible place so I can always review them, and my pain levels, current obstacles, moods, and feelings are regularly and openly addressed.

My doctors overlap in care, agree with one personalized treatment plan, and work to educate me and positively impact the outcome of my health. With each appointment, I gain valuable insight, am given skilled consideration, and have a reason to have confidence in my care.

Of all the reasons to be traveling on this plane, mine is medical, and I can guess that I am a minority in this sea of business travelers around me. I have completed eight years of these prescheduled out-of-state cancer hospital appointments. Traveling back and forth, I have met many brave people who did not accept the limited prognosis given to them, made a change in their care providers, and are now beating all the odds that were once against them.

Back and forth I go, as many times as my team requests that I be here. My sleep begins to suffer as the date approaches, and my subconscious fills with anxiety as I prepare again to face the intense days of back-to-back appointments on my long itinerary. I do not always recognize the looming stress as it approaches. I could not even stop it if I knew. It is a buried thought that hides in my mind and wakes me up as I try to process what I know and prepare for what I do not know. Somewhere in my mind, it has taken up residence, and I am surprised by the rights it still has after so many years.

Again, I feel slight while lying on the exam table in the threadbare hospital gown, waiting for the exam to begin. I admire this out-of-state oncologist. He always personalizes these appointments and gives me the prognosis in a straightforward manner, which is why, when I found him, no other substitute would suffice.

He carries an air of confidence, seriousness, and gentleness as he enters the room. He always remembers me and appears to have considered my circumstances long before I arrived. I trust him, his thirty years of experience, his maturity, and his wisdom. Holding my chart in his hand, he is well-versed in every aspect of the tumor and never takes up our appointment time reading the folder of notes in front of him.

Two years after my hysterectomy, this same doctor told me during a routine appointment that there had been a better way. "We would have never done the surgery," he boldly said, directed at his accompanying nurse practitioner in the room, who nodded in agreement. "We would have put you on a medication to suppress your ovaries and then observed you to see if those cells grew."

What? There was another way? There was nowhere in my brain to hold that response and alternate possibilities. I just heard clearly that my organs never needed to be eliminated, and I was once again astonished. I felt ignorant, damaged, rushed along, and tricked. Somebody should have explained these things to me years ago until I understood all my options. Since the hysterectomy, I had had years of remorse and ongoing troubleshooting to navigate the repercussions that it has had on my health and emotional well-being.

It is easy to deduce why I travel to this hospital, and I am always grateful to finally arrive and be in front of such watchful, skilled eyes. There are pages of stats, levels being checked, and components in blood of which I have never heard. These are referred to as "cancer markers," and I remain amazed because that term signifies that this whole thing could have been detected before it ever started.

"It's not coming back," the doctor said definitively and unexpectedly without mincing words as he completed the exam. He had decreed his very educated, very well-considered opinion, and it was over. Finalized in a moment, it shifted my thinking just as on the day I learned about the tumor. It was so unexpected and sudden that I had to ask if he really said what he just said.

He explained that he was assured, and he made the space to help me realize that I could also be assured. I could stop bracing for these appointments and stop waiting and needing his all clear. I had walked it out and done all the necessary things on this journey. I could let my guard down and entirely choose hope, with permission. I believed him. We had finished this dance, and

I could now move on from this looming cliff where I existed in thought for a season.

With all the uncertainties of cancer and reasons to remain braced for the worst, I now choose hope. I have a shield of hope that has taken me ten years to steady, faithfully using wisdom and skill. I hold up that shield to any and every thought that tells me this is not over, that the cancer could come back, and that it will not end well.

My belief is now stronger than my fear, my anxiety, and the stress that it is so commonly partnered with. Cancer came and went, and I am still standing here, the same wife, mother, daughter, and grandma, the same person I was before this started, only stronger. Cancer has no power and no control, and I am no longer fearful.

RESTORATION

This chapter is the most sentimental of all for me to write. I have realized that to understand the blessing from a trial is to trust the great purpose on the other side of the pain. I have never abandoned God's plan, although there were days when I wondered if I had. Amid the battle, often none of it made sense. I could not understand why I was going through this or what positive things could come out of it, but still some did.

On one of my hospital visits during the first few years of treatments, I grabbed a complimentary hat from a basket at the check-in counter during an appointment. It was a lavender-colored knit hat and was a gift graciously made and donated by a women's church group. I imagined them sitting around and offering their skills, and I found it a heartfelt reminder that there were people out there who cared a great deal about strangers.

Until then, I had not worn many hats, but these felt warm and soft, and I appreciated that someone cared enough to make them. I grabbed the package as a reminder, but I also wondered if there would be a time when I needed that hat or if I felt I could go out in public with just that on my bald head. But I could not, and I never did. So, the hat remained in its plastic bag, and I kept it for years, always mindlessly burying it in my sock drawer for no real reason.

My sister stated clearly, early on that there was no decision to make when considering whether to follow the doctor's care plan. Having worked in the medical field, she had a natural draw to medicine and a trust in doctors that I never had the opportunity to develop. She summed up our brief conversation on the topic with, "Don't you want to see your grandkids one day?"

Those were heavy words for me since I had spent my career working with children, and I clearly valued and looked forward to having my own grandchildren one day. She knew how to make her point, and since I had no other direction or better plan, I followed along, doing everything expected of me without rebuttal. At the time, there was no scenario even close to hinting of grandchildren in my future, but I chose not to argue and accepted that logic.

Five years and a lot of family life later, we welcomed our first grandchild, a little girl. She was an absolute treasure from the moment she was born and a bright light in every day we spent together. Feeling that I was mostly back to my old self, I spent most of my days caring for her. She and I had many adventures together, dancing, reading, singing, and walking in the neighborhood. She brought so much joy every day to my life; even her name translated means joy. She was and is still a gift and a blessing, and I had no idea of all that she would restore to my life.

She loved our days together, walking through the neighborhood, noticing every dog, and trying to engage every person who smiled at her along the way. There was a big water fountain in the town square, and I would unbuckle her from her seat for a moment so that she could get out of the stroller and put her hands in the water. She was filled with energy, climbing on everything with boundless spurts and running across the green spaces, faster and faster, as I ran behind her. I loved every minute of it. She was daring, bold, sweet, intelligent, and full of personality. We spent many days together, filled with endless fun.

I wanted to take my granddaughter for a stroller ride one fall day, but the afternoon had grown unexpectedly chilly and windy. Wanting to dress her warmer than the coat she had come over in, I buckled her in the seat, bundled her in a blanket, and then remembered the lavender hat. I grabbed it from the bottom of my sock bin, unwrapped it, and placed it on her head. She immediately liked it and accepted it as her own. It fit her perfectly, covering her head down to her big brown eyes.

She wore that hat proudly that day as if it had always been hers and continued to do so many days later. Some days, she would go home in the hat and show up in it again the next day. She insisted on wearing it indoors and outdoors and sometimes even sleeping in the hat at night. The hat had found its rightful owner, and I was touched remembering the circumstances and where it came from.

One day, I was talking with my daughter-in-law and mentioned how often my grandbaby wore the hat. I told her the hat story—how I had never worn it but saved it all those years and how I thought it was remarkable how much she loved it. In a very matter-of-fact response, and without hesitation, my daughter-in-law said, "Look at God's promise coming full circle." Of course it was God's promise. How had I missed that? My granddaughter was God's promise, and this was full circle.

God had always intended that hat for her. God wanted me to recognize His promise coming to pass. Five years before, when I grabbed that hat in the middle of my desperate circumstances, God was in the middle of a bigger plan. There was another, much happier season on the way, part of a bigger story, that I could not see at the time.

Now, I have a second grandchild, a little girl, and another

promise that I had no idea would bring such joy with her endless hugs, sweet smiles, and playfulness. I also see her daily, and she beams with new life and has a unique little personality all her own. Because of her, I was now sitting in a room at a small Saturday evening church service. We had gathered to witness this new baby being dedicated to God by her parents.

As our extended family sprawled across a row, we heard a message about saying yes to what God asks you to do. Across the screen, written in bold letters, was a clear directive: "Write the story, tell the tale, sing the song, because you cannot know who and everyone who might need to hear it." I pulled back multiple times in many seasons, not knowing how to finish a chapter or formulate an idea within these pages. I found help and hope in documenting my journey to share, and that reporting had now led me here. And yes, I would write the book.

I did not want to finish my life with regrets, and I did not want to miss anyone who needed to hear this story. Ultimately, it was not about what I might say wrong but whom I might reach with what I did say.

That is why I am here, having survived cancer with enough drive and perseverance to encourage the next person to believe that their story is not over either. God truly is the author and finisher of our faith, the beginning and the end, our ever-present help in times of need, and the One who knows every part of us. It is OK to struggle, weaken, fall, and succumb for the moment. But you do not have to stay down or in that low place, because you are never alone.

Faith identifies us and connects us when we believe. He promises that we can be whole, finish strong, and be victorious on this earth and in heaven. I believe that, and I am living it out. I must because there is no other conclusion I can draw that makes sense of the facts and carefully connects all the details to that one magnificent picture.

Life has moved on for me since my breast cancer diagnosis in 2014. It flowed naturally with graduations, moves, new homes, weddings, births, and career changes. I now operate a small preschool, allowing my husband and me to care for our grandchildren and other children from the community.

Our house radiates with the sounds of joy from little children partaking in life, something I could not know would be part of the picture from the beginning of this story. The connections, plans, purpose, and destiny I witness are indescribably evident and worth every challenge. Yes, there was pain, but understanding the purpose of the pain defines the journey. In peace, I confidently profess that it is well with my soul.

SINCERELY

Dear Friend,

I am sharing this with you today not because I want to, but because I need to. This new cancer diagnosis has forced me into a place I did not see coming. It feels like the great segregator between me and the rest of the world. I am dealing with something I spend the day trying to think through, understand, and come to terms with. I am doing all I can to understand the information, the medications, the diagnosis, the treatments, the options, and anything else my sources refrained from telling me or may not have known.

Right now, my days are filled with what-if questions that I am trying to sort out in whatever little time I have that is not already filled. The appointments, phone calls, test results, and endless waiting consumes every day. I often must share this information, and I am left to console those I share it with. To say I am overwhelmed is a large understatement.

People, in their care and concern, try their best to figure out how to help or console me. I want to take this opportunity to express what really does help. Please know that when you see me there is a lot going on in my mind. Right now, you cannot fix it or change that for me. Statistics you heard, unsolicited advice, or the story of anyone else's experience does not help. I am walking through an unknown place that can feel very dark and lonely. Like I said, it is the great segregator, only not very great.

I am most supported when you listen more than you advise and extend grace to me if I seem distracted. I am doing my best to focus on some normal parts of my life, but it takes new energy, and I am tired and at times depleted. I spend my days mentally and emotionally challenged. I am on a journey, and I have no idea what the conclusion will be. I must walk it out, and I need the space and opportunity to do that.

Nobody else has an experience that can or will be mine. I want my normal life back, and when you see me trying to get that, it is not because I am pretending nothing is wrong but because, instead, I am trying to find a new balance with all that is on this new plate. When I am ready to talk, it is easier for me to share in a place with no judgment, opinions, or well-intended advice. When I share even a small piece right now, it is because it feels big to me. Please listen and try to understand that to me there is no part of this that is insignificant.

Any method that you want to connect with me right now is helpful, even if I do not have the energy to express this fact very well. I will never forget that you reached out and did something to try to connect with me in my pain. It will all mean a lot and more than you will ever know. When I look back on this time, I will see that it was your caring gestures that reminded me, supported me, and gave me strength to cope. I promise that your understanding and listening speaks volumes and helps.

Please know that everywhere I go, I bring an elephant that sits in the room with me. Many times, it is too hard for me to look at or acknowledge, but when I have the strength and I am ready to, please accept whatever that looks like without judgment.

Remember that I did not ask for or choose this, but if you ever need me to understand what you might need in the same situation, I now have a small idea of what that looks like.

Sincerely,
A cancer patient

Conclusion

It is a Sunday, and it is approaching ten years since the start of my cancer journey. Sitting here in the library with less tangible goals than to complete this book on any respectable timeline, I am still amazed at all that this journey included and what it turned out to be. I am wrapping up the content, double-checking the punctuation, and rereading some of my most impactful memories.

Looking around and pondering some of the thoughts I have tried to relate on these pages, I looked up on the wall to find an incredibly impactful quote that explains why I started this project: "No one with books is ever alone, even in the darkest moments." That was written by the author Rachel Caine, and it summarizes my purpose and hope for every reader. If you have felt alone facing cancer, I hope that in reading this, you will feel partnered with, understood, and appreciated by others all around you. We are in the same fight with you and rooting for your victory despite every mounding obstacle and setback you face.

God inspired the title of this book in the very first moments when I began to feel led to write it. I had never attempted a writing project and wrote out everything that came to my mind. I did not understand at the time all that the title would inspire. But then the season came when I had the motivation and the vison to tell the story that went along with the title.

As I recalled the events, the emotions, and the timelines, it helped me see and unpack the issues surrounding my identity, loss, and direction. When I began to sort through and unload the feelings that went with the diagnosis and the path I had taken, healing began to happen. Surprisingly, the raw emotions were still very present in the memories even after years had passed. God always knows the title of all our stories and the contents of every one of our chapters. Greatness, inspiration, value, and purpose are in each of us. Everyone has a story that could help someone else if they were to hear it.

Over the years, I had often forgotten about or talked myself out of finishing *My Pink Choice*. I had never considered all that my story was before beginning to document my experience with cancer. *Maybe the cancer will come back and there will be a new cancer chapter,* I hesitantly thought. *Maybe* My Pink Choice *will mean that I did not choose the treatments the second time and that my choice was not viable, and then the story will not end well. What if nobody wants to read this or can connect to or understand the need to discuss and consider what a cancer diagnosis feels like? What if the purpose I intended gets lost in the final product?*

Once I understood who God was for me in this situation, I decided to follow a path of faith. It was not easy or without unexpected challenges. Everyone faces obstacles, fears, and moments of desperation. It is a commission to learn to carry those burdens, leaning on a loving God who is committed to sharing them with you. I turned to God as I worked through struggles, remaining close to Him when every other method failed. I found freedom as I made that choice and relinquished control over my circumstances. I prayed continuously for spiritual light to come into every dark place in my life.

Cancer and the season around me were dark, but light came in everywhere as I learned to trust God. That is the beautiful thing about light: once it illuminates the darkness, you cannot unsee what is there. I have admittedly struggled with so many parts of this journey, but I have also witnessed the peace, the justice, and the recompense that comes from choosing faith and trusting God with the life He gave me.

God knows, cares, and always has had a good plan for me that often I could not see.

Sometimes, sadness, trauma, or loss overtakes us in our circumstances. Other times, we push along, barely realizing the need to include God in our everyday lives. We recognize God was the closest in the challenges, the hopelessness, and the pain. He longs to be the catalyst for our strength, courage, and redemption when we choose to rely on Him to play that role.

I hope this story reminds you that God is also with you in every trial and is yours in completeness, surrender, and sacrifice. You are not alone. He is ready to meet you in the hardest struggles and rescue you from your desperation. Despite what you may have been told, there is nothing missing or broken about you in the eyes of your loving Father in heaven who created you.

I now understand that I have reached the conclusion of so many processes in this trial, and what remains has added immense value to my life. I have discovered a faith that overpowered the darkness and brought joy to my spirit. Not every trial and turn were easy or good, but I learned something valuable from each of them. I can confidently draft the story, confront the adversity, and arrive at a conclusion with hope and purpose. I have unshakable confidence in God that I never owned before in this journey, and there is satisfaction in knowing that this ending is good.

Be well and live your life fully with unapologetic faith, knowing you are being held in God's loving arms.

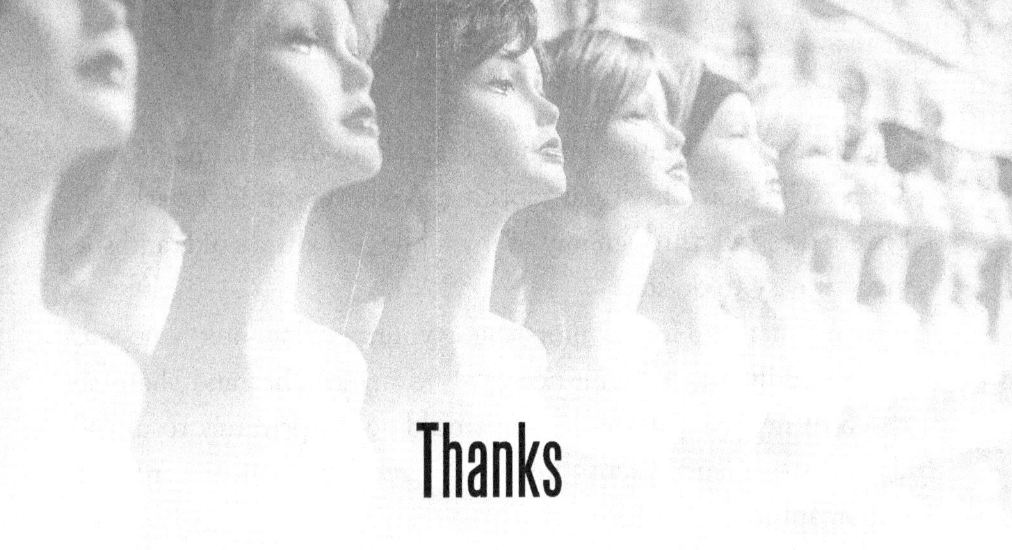

Thanks

I am grateful to my husband for steadying me in my desperation, stabilizing me when the ground shifted, and never leaving me alone. He never considered giving up and has remained the anchor I always needed. Every time I looked over, he was standing by my side, holding everything I no longer wanted to carry (my purse and my burdens). Years later, I still find him holding my hand, holding me up, closely tracking my health, and gathering multiple supplements every night to hand to me on a schedule.

I am so thankful for my son, who sincerely and repeatedly asked me, "Mom, how are you doing?" and then really listened while I answered. He pointed to the truth in the middle of my circumstances, prayed earnestly, and found ways to make me laugh frequently. I am grateful that he and I could share humor during stressful moments and pray when God said to pray. I am grateful for his love and compassion shared freely during this season and for changing my outcome with his faith.

I appreciate my daughter, who has always been deeply invested. As a personal confidant, closet editor, and faithful friend, she tirelessly cheered me on, encouraged me to keep going, and believed in the outcome whenever I gave up. Her belief and encouragement fueled this project through many seasons. I will never forget when she carefully asked me how I felt about discovering my new lopsided look on Christmas morning. And every time she asked if I needed to talk through any of my feelings. I always did, and she made it easy to do so.

I am thankful for my empathetic youngest daughter, who was extra cuddly and felt the need to see my stitches and share so much of my pain firsthand. We would go off privately to unveil the bandages and discuss her tender feelings, which were also important moments for me.

I am grateful for my optimistic but serious middle girl, who overthinks asking questions and then thinks long and hard, choosing her encouraging words carefully. I have saved every sentimental, thoughtful note and picture that she used to express her young feelings in that season.

I am grateful for my daughter-in-law and grandchildren, who inspired me and are my beautiful promises of God on the other side of this mountain. They resonate with joy and have been worth going through every ugly, dark battle to meet them on the other side. I proudly call them mine and cannot imagine my world without the love and hope they regularly fill my life with.

I am thankful for my family, who faced the illness with support and concern, navigating the weakness, hair loss, and food challenges as my unexpected news interrupted everyone's life. They picked up the slack, made up for the lack, and rallied in the moments that would have been so much harder had they not shown up to care.

I am grateful to my closest friends who kept calling to check in. I am aware those were hard phone calls to make—calls without a personal agenda, giving me the time and space to share openly and emotionally, without judgment or unsolicited advice. Each was a lifeline across the miles I desperately needed and will always treasure.

I am thankful for my female coworkers who stopped by my desk and told me that my short, dark, curly hair was cute. It was not cute to me, but I appreciated their time in convincing me. Their friendship and caring outweighed my struggle at that moment.

I am also thankful for the numerous women I have encountered who unselfishly shared their stories and unknowingly inspired me to write mine. They were strong, courageous, transparent, and inspiring in attitude and perseverance. I bless each one with the strength they imparted to me.

I remember those who accompanied me to my appointments, distracted me, and made the trip, the long days, and the daunting schedule memorable for a happy reason. Two are always better than one. Thanks for being there.

I am grateful for the motherly nurse who hugged me after my biopsy and genuinely told me everything would be OK. Her sincerity carried me in those early moments as I believed her and clung to what she said.

I remember fondly the nonprofit organizations that sent gas cards and hats, paid a bill, wrote a note, and interrupted my stress with their care. I cherished those connections and have saved every life-giving note.

Printed in the United States
by Baker & Taylor Publisher Services